Rapid Paediatrics and Child Health

RAPID PAEDIATRICS AND CHILD HEALTH

Helen Brough
Rola Alkurdi
Ram Nataraja
All of
Royal Free and University College Medical School,
University College London, London
Ajenthan Surendranathan
St Bartholomew's and the London Hospital, London

EDITORIAL ADVISORS
Brent Taylor
Professor of Community Child Health,
Royal Free and University College Medical School,
University College London, London
Alastair Sutcliffe
Senior Lecturer in Paediatrics
Royal Free and University College Medical School,
University College London, London

SERIES EDITOR
Amir H. Sam
Royal Free and University College Medical School,
University College London, London

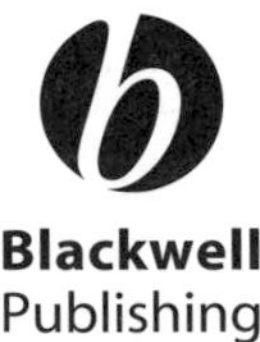

Blackwell
Publishing

Published by Blackwell Publishing Ltd
Blackwell Publishing, Inc., 350 Main Street, Malden,
Massachusetts 02148-5020, USA
Blackwell Publishing Ltd, 9600 Garsington Road, Oxford OX4 2DQ, UK
Blackwell Publishing Asia Pty Ltd, 550 Swanston Street, Carlton,
Victoria 3053, Australia

First published 2004

Library of Congress Cataloging-in-Publication Data

Rapid paediatrics / Helen Brough ... [et al.].
p. ; cm. – (Rapid series)
Includes bibliographical references.
ISBN 1-4051-1642-0 (alk. paper)
1. Pediatrics–Handbooks, manuals, etc.
[DNLM: 1. Pediatrics–Handbooks. WS 39 R218 2004] I. Brough, Helen. II. Series.

RJ48.R375 2004
618.92–dc22

2004002496

ISBN 1-4051-1642-0

A catalogue record for this title is available from the British Library

Set in Frutiger 7/9pt
by Kolam Information Services Pvt. Ltd, Pondicherry, India
Printed and bound in India by Replika Press Pvt. Ltd

Commissioning Editor: Vicki Noyes
Editorial Assistant: Nicola Ulyatt
Production Editor: Lorna Hind
Production Controller: Kate Charman

For further information on Blackwell Publishing, visit our website:
http://www.blackwellpublishing.com

The publisher's policy is to use permanent paper from mills that operate a sustainable forestry policy, and which has been manufactured from pulp processed using acid-free and elementary chlorine-free practices. Furthermore, the publisher ensures that the text paper and cover board used have met acceptable environmental accreditation standards.

Contents

Foreword

Rapid Paediatrics and Child Health has been written by a group of able prize-winning clinical medical students from the Royal Free and University College Medical School. They have developed a system that facilitates understanding of paediatric conditions, most of them common and all of those included, important. The authors have achieved an excellent synthesis that should help in the care of individual children, while maintaining a population and social perspective. This is a refreshing textbook that will allow rapid and thorough review of paediatrics and child health.

London
January 2004

Brent Taylor
Professor of Community Child Health

Alastair Sutcliffe
Senior Lecturer in Paediatrics

Preface

Rapid Paediatrics and Child Health is part of a series of books for medical students that are designed to facilitate learning about core topics in a structured format. Each page is divided into our own 'surgical sieve': Definition, Aetiology, Association/Risk factors, Epidemiology, History, Examination, Pathology/Pathophysiology, Investigations, Management, Complications, and Prognosis. In this book we have included over 150 topics that cover major topics in all paediatric specialities and neonatology. We have included core knowledge as well as up-to-date national guidelines, important new investigative techniques, and treatment options. The investigations mentioned are by no means carried out in all children with a certain condition but only if they are deemed necessary. This book has been designed to be easy to carry around and to allow rapid access to information when in clinic or on wards so that you can consolidate theory with practice. We hope you enjoy reading this book as much as we have enjoyed writing it!

Our editorial advisors Professor Brent Taylor and Dr Alastair Sutcliffe have been a fantastic support and we are very grateful for the hours they have put in to making this book possible. We would also like to thank Dr Giles Kendall, who kindly reviewed our neonatal topics.

London
January 2004

Helen Brough
Rola Alkurdi
Ram Nataraja
Ajenthan Surendranathan

ABC airway, breathing, circulation
ABG arterial blood gases
ABVD adriamycin, bleomycin, vinblastine, and dacarbazine
ACTH adrenocorticotrophic hormone
AD autosomal dominant
ADHD attention deficit hyperactivity disorder
AFP alpha fetoprotein
AIDS acquired immunodeficiency syndrome
ALL acute lymphoblastic leukaemia
ALP alkaline phosphatase
ALT alanine aminotransferase
ALTE apparent life-threatening event
AML acute myeloblastic leukaemia
AN anorexia nervosa
AP anteroposterior
APTT activated partial thromboplastin time
AR aortic regurgitation
AR autosomal recessive
ARDS acute respiratory distress syndrome
ARF acute renal failure
ASA aminosalicylic acid
ASD atrial septal defect
ASOT anti-streptolysin O titre
AST aspartate aminotransferase
ATG antithymocyte globulin
ATN acute tubular necrosis
ATP adenosine triphosphate
AV atrioventricular
AVPU alert, verbal response, painful response, unresponsive
AVSD atrioventricular septal defect
AXR abdominal X-ray
b.d. twice a day
BCG bacille Calmette–Guérin
BiPAP bilevel positive airways pressure
BM blood monitor/monitoring
BMD Becker muscular dystrophy
BMI body mass index
BMJ *British Medical Journal*
BMT bone marrow transplant/transplantation
BP blood pressure
BPD bronchopulmonary dysplasia
bpm beat per minute
BTS British Thoracic Society
CAD coronary artery disease
cAMP cyclic adenosine monophosphatase
CBT cognitive–behavioural therapy
CCDC consultant in communicable disease control
CD Crohn's disease
CDH congenital diaphragmatic hernia
CF cystic fibrosis
CFTR cystic fibrosis transmembrane regulator
CGG cytosine-guanine-guanine
CHB complete heart block
CHD congenital heart disease
CHF congestive heart failure
CLD chronic lung disease
CMV cytomegalovirus
CNS central nervous system
COA coarctation of the aorta
CPAP continuous positive airways pressure
CPK creatinine phosphokinase
CRF chronic renal failure
CRHD chronic rheumatic heart disease
CRP C-reactive protein
CSF cerebrospinal fluid
CT computerised tomography
CTG cardiotocography/graph
CVP central venous pressure
CVS chorionic villous sampling
CXR chest X-ray/radiograph
DD differential diagnosis
DDH developmental dysplasia of the hip
DDT dichlorodiphenyltri-chloroethane

List of abbreviations

DEXA	dual-energy X-ray absorptiometry
DIC	disseminated intravascular coagulation/coagulopathy
DIP	distal intraphalangeal
DISIDA	diisopropyl iminodiacetic acid
DKA	diabetic ketoacidosis
DM	diabetes mellitus
DMD	Duchenne muscular dystrophy
DMPK	dystrophia myotonica protein kinase
DMSA	dimercaptosuccinic acid
DNA	deoxyribonucleic acid
DNAse	deoxyribonuclease
DPT	diphtheria, pertussis, tetanus
DSM-IV	*Diagnostic and Statistical Manual of Mental Disorders*, 4th edition
DTPA	diethylenetriamine pentaacetic acid
DVT	deep vein thrombosis
EBV	Epstein–Barr virus
ECG	electrocardiogram/graph
ECMO	extracorporeal membrane oxygenation
EEG	electroencephalogram
ELISA	enzyme-linked immunosorbent assay
EMG	electromyogram/graph
ENT	ear nose throat
EPO	erythropoietin
ERCP	endoscopic retrograde cholangiopan-creatography
ESR	erythrocyte sedimentation rate
ET	endotracheal
FVIII–FXI	factor VIII to factor XI
FAB	French–American–British
FAS	foetal alcohol syndrome
FBC	full blood count
FEV	forced expiratory volume
FFP	fresh frozen plasma
FGFR3	fibroblast growth factor receptor 3
FH	father's height (cm)
FMR1	fragile-X mental retardation 1
FMRP	fragile-X mental retardation protein
FSH	follicle-stimulating hormone
G6PD	glucose-6-phosphate dehydrogenase
GBS	group B streptococcus
GCS	graduated compression stockings
GFR	glomerular filtration rate
GH	growth hormone
GI	gastrointestinal
GN	glomerulonephritis
GnRH	gonadotrophin-releasing hormone
GOR	gastro-oesophageal reflux
GORD	gastro-oesophageal reflux disease
GP	general practitioner
GSD	glycogen storage disease
GTCS	generalised tonic-clonic seizures
GU	genitourinary
GVHD	graft-versus-host disease
HA	haemophilia A
HAV	Hepatitis A virus
Hb	haemoglobin
HB	haemophilia B
HBV	hepatitis B virus
HC	haemophilia C
HCG	human chorionic gonadotrophin
HCV	hepatitis C virus
HDL	high-density lipoprotein
HFO	high frequency oscillation
Hib	*Haemophilus influenzae* b

HIDA	hepatobiliary iminodiacetic acid
HIE	hypoxic–ischaemic encephalopathy
His	histidine
HIV	human immunodeficiency virus
HLA	human lymphocyte antigen
HR	heart rate
HS	hereditary spherocytosis
HSP	Henoch–Schönlein purpura
HSV	herpes simplex virus
HTLV	human T-lymphotropic virus
HUS	haemolytic uraemic syndrome
IBS	irritable bowel syndrome
ICP	intracranial pressure
ICS	inhaled corticosteroids
ICSI	intracytoplasmic sperm injection
ICU	intensive care unit
Ig	immunoglobulin
IGFBP-3	insulin-like growth factor–binding protein 3
IHD	ischaemic heart disease
INR	international normalised ratio
IM	intramuscular
IP	intraphalangeal
IUGR	intrauterine growth restriction/retardation
IV	intravenous
IVH	intraventricular haemorrhage
IVU	intravenous urogram
JVP	jugular venous pulse
LABA	long-acting β_2-agonist
LCPD	Legg–Calvé–Perthes disease
LDH	lactate dehydrogenase
LFT	liver function test
LGA	large for gestational age
LH	luteinising hormone
LHRH	luteinising-hormone-releasing hormone
LIF	left iliac fossa
LP	lumbar puncture
LRTI	lower respiratory tract infection
LVF	left ventricular function
LVH	left ventricular hypertrophy
MAG3	mercaptoacetyltri-glycine
MALT	mucosa-associated lymphoid tissue
MCH	mean cell/corpuscular haemoglobin
MC+S	microscopy culture + sensitivity
MCUG	micturating cystourethrogram
MCV	mean cell/corpuscular volume
MDD	major depressive disorder
Men C	meningitis C
MH	mother's height (cm)
MMR	measles, mumps, rubella
MR	mitral regurgitation
MRI	magnetic resonance imaging
MSE	mental state examination
MSU	midstream specimen of urine
MVP	mitral valve prolapse
NA	noradrenaline
NAI	nonaccidental injury
NBM	nucleus basalis magnocellularis
NEC	necrotising enterocolitis
NEJM	*New England Journal of Medicine*
NF	neurofibromatosis
NG	nasogastric
NHL	non-Hodgkin's lymphoma
NICE	National Institute for Consumer Education
NICU	neonatal intensive care unit
NK	natural killer
NO	nitric oxide
NSAID	nonsteroidal anti-inflammatory drug
NSPCC	National Society for the Prevention of Cruelty to Children
OCA	oculocutaneous albinism

List of abbreviations

OCD	obsessive–compulsive disorder
OCP	oral contraceptive pill
OGD	oesophagogastroduodenoscopy
OPV	oral polio vaccine
ORT	oral rehydration therapy
OTC	over-the-counter
PA	pulmonary artery
PAS	periodic acid–Schiff
PCP	*Pneumocystis carinii* pneumonia
PCR	polymerase chain reaction
PDA	patent ductus arteriosus
PE	pulmonary embolism
PEN	pharmacy equivalent name
PET	positron emission tomography
PICU	paediatric intensive care unit
PKU	phenylketonuria
PNH	paroxysmal nocturnal haemoglobinuria
p.o.	per os
POS	polycystic ovary syndrome
PPH	persistent pulmonary hypertension
PPV	positive pressure ventilation
PROM	prolonged rupture of membranes
PSC	primary sclerosing cholangitis
PTH	parathyroid hormone
PTSD	post-traumatic stress disorder
PUVA	psoralen ultraviolet A
q.d.s.	four times a day
RAH	right atrial hypertrophy
RBC	red blood cell/count
RDS	respiratory distress syndrome
REAL	revised European and American lymphoma
REM	rapid eye movement
Rh	rhesus
rhGH	recombinant human growth hormone
RIF	right iliac fossa
RNA	ribonucleic acid
ROM	range of movement
ROP	retinopathy of prematurity
RSV	respiratory syncitial virus
RTA	road traffic accident
RVH	right ventricular hypertrophy
RVT	renal vein thrombosis
SBP	systolic blood pressure
SC	subcutaneous
SCBU	Special Care Baby Unit
SCID	severe combined immunodeficiency
S/E	side-effects
SGA	small for gestational age
SIADH	syndrome of inappropriate antidiuretic hormone
SIDS	sudden infant death syndrome
SIgAD	selective immunoglobulin A deficiency
SIRS	systemic inflammatory response syndrome
SLE	systemic lupus erythematosus
SMA	superior mesenteric artery
SOB	shortness of breath
SPAG	small particle aerosol generation
SSPE	subacute sclerosing panencephalitis
SSRI	selective serotonin reuptake inhibitor
STD	sexually transmitted disease
SUDEP	sudden unexpected death in epileptic patients
SUFE	slipped upper femoral epiphysis
SVC	superior vena cava
SVT	supraventricular tachycardia
SW	southwest
T_3	tri-iodothyronine
T_4	thyroxine
TB	tuberculosis
t.d.s.	three times a day
TFT	thyroid function test

TGA	transposition of the great arteries
THAM	tris(hydroxymethyl)-aminomethane
TLC	total lung capacity
TOF	tracheo-oesophageal fistula
TOP	termination of pregnancy
TORCH	toxoplasma, other (syphilis, HIV), rubella, cytomegalovirus, hepatitis
TPN	total parenteral nutrition
TRH	thyrotropin-releasing hormone
TS	transient synovitis
TS1&2	tuberous sclerosis 1&2
TSH	thyroid-stimulating hormone
TSI	thyroid-stimulating immunoglobulin
TSS	toxic shock syndrome
TTN	transient tachypnoea of the newborn
TTP	thrombotic thrombocytopenic purpura
U&E	urea and electrolytes
UC	ulcerative colitis
UDPGA	uridine diphosphoglucuronic acid
UKALL	United Kingdom Medical Research Council protocol for childhood ALL
URT	upper respiratory tract
URTI	upper respiratory tract infection
USS	ultrasound scan
UTI	urinary tract infection
UTR	untranslated region
UV	ultraviolet
VACTERL	vertebral, anal, cardiac, tracheal, esophageal, renal, limb
VE	varicella embryopathy
VF	ventricular fibrillator
VON	varicella of the newborn
VSD	ventricular septal defect
VT	ventricular tachycardia
VUR	vesicoureteric reflux
VZV	varicella zoster virus
WCC	white cell count
WHO	World Health Organization
WPW	Wolff–Parkinson–White (syndrome)
XLA	X-linked agammaglobulinaemia
F	female
M	male
1°	primary
2°	secondary
↑	increase(d)
↓	decrease(d)
→	to/lead(s) to
>	greater than
<	less than
~	approximately
×	times

Rapid series mnemonic

D:	Definition	Doctors
A:	Aetiology	Are
A/R:	Associations/Risk factors	Always
E:	Epidemiology	Emphasising
H:	History	History-taking &
E:	Examination	Examining
P:	Pathology	Patients
I:	Investigations	In
M:	Management	Managing
C:	Complications	Clinical
P:	Prognosis	Problems

CONDITIONS

D: **SGA:** birth weight < 20th percentile for gestational age or < 2.5 kg.
LGA: birth weight > 90th percentile for gestational age or > 4 kg.

A: **SGA:** may be familial, constitutional, or due to IUGR.
IUGR is defined as either symmetrical or asymmetrical:
Asymmetrical IUGR: relative sparing of head circumference in relation to weight and length:

- Due to impaired uteroplacental function 2° to maternal pre-eclampsia, DM or nutritional deficiency during the 3rd trimester.
- Occurs when foetal growth rate in 3rd trimester exceeds maximal supply from the placenta.
- There is preferential sparing of the cerebral perfusion at times of foetal distress.

Symmetrical IUGR: head circumference, weight, and length are all proportionally affected to equivalent degrees:

- Indicative of a prolonged period of poor intrauterine growth.
- Caused by congenital intrauterine infections (TORCH) in the 1st trimester, genetic factors such as single gene deletions and chromosomal disorders, maternal smoking, drug and alcohol abuse, chronic medical conditions (e.g. CRF), malnutrition, or multiple pregnancies.

LGA: macrosomia is a feature of infants of mothers with either gestational or poorly controlled/undiagnosed DM.

A/R: **IUGR:** previous SGA infant, low pre-pregnancy weight and poor pregnancy weight gain.

E: **SGA:** affects by definition 20% of the population and varies with ethnic background.
IUGR: 2/200 neonates; asymmetrical > symmetrical IUGR.
LGA: affects by definition 20% of live births; is more common in developed countries where there is a higher prevalence of DM.

H&E: **Antenatal:** maternal examination and accurate dating aid diagnosis. Oligohydramnios and poor foetal movements are indications of placental insufficiency.
Perinatal monitoring: foetal tachycardia, loss of variability of the baseline in the foetal heart trace, and late decelerations may indicate foetal distress on CTG.
Postnatal measurements: birth weight, length, and head circumference on centile chart.

P: See **A**.

I: **Radiology:** USS is the 1° method of diagnosing IUGR or macrosomia antenatally.
Cordocentesis: percutaneous umbilical blood sampling may be used for detection of hypoxia, lactic acidosis, hypoglycaemia, chromosomal analysis, and DNA diagnosis of congenital intrauterine infections.

M: **Antenatal:** maternal bedrest and limitation of activity for severe IUGR.
Perinatal: maternal administration of O_2, continuous assessment of foetal well-being.
Delivery (IUGR): if foetus becomes hypoxic *in utero*, an emergency Caesarean section is required.
Macrosomia: induce at 38/40 to prevent complications in a unit with good neonatal facilities.

C: **IUGR foetus:** intrauterine hypoxia, birth asphyxia, and death.
IUGR infant: hypothermia (relatively large surface area), hypoglycaemia (poor fat and glycogen stores), hypocalcaemia, polycythaemia, and meconium aspiration.
LGA: birth asphyxia due to prolonged/difficult delivery, birth trauma, especially shoulder dystocia, hypoglycaemia in the neonatal period due to hyperinsulinism, and polycythaemia.

P: Depends on the cause of abnormal size at birth. Infants with asymmetrical IUGR will rapidly put on weight in the postnatal period; symmetrical IUGR infants are more likely to remain small permanently. Studies have shown that IUGR infants are at ↑risk of developing ↑BP, Type II DM, and coronary heart disease.

D: Inflammation of the pilosebaceous duct. Classified as mild, moderate, and severe.

A: **Adolescent acne:**

- ↑Sebum production: androgenic stimulation of hyper-responsive pilosebaceous units.
- Impaired normal flow of sebum: obstruction of the pilosebaceous duct by hyperkeratosis.
- Propioni acne bacteria: may play a role by producing cytokines and lipolytic enzymes.

Infantile acne: <3 months of life; transient and usually due to maternal androgens.

A/R: Puberty, may ↑ premenstrually, POS, excess cortisol (Cushing syndrome).

E: **Developed world:** affects 79–95% of the adolescent population, peaking at 14–18 years; tends to recede by early twenties.
Developing world: acne incidence is considerably lower; likely combination of environmental and genetic factors.

H: Usually self-diagnosed, acute onset, greasy skin, may be painful.

E: **Open comedones:** whiteheads; flesh-coloured papules.
Closed comedones: blackheads; black colour is due to oxidation of the melanin pigment.
Other features: pustules, nodules, cysts, scarring, and seborrhoea.
Distribution: primarily affects the face, neck, chest, and back (where sebaceous glands are most numerous).

P: Gross distension of the pilosebaceous follicle with neutrophil infiltration. Closed comedones may contain serous fluid. Severe acne can create fistulae between inflamed glands.

I: Normally none required. Investigate for endocrine disorder if acne develops during 2–10 years of age.
Bloods: FSH, LH (if female, suspect POS).
Urine: 24-h-urinary cortisol (if Cushing syndrome is suspected).

M: Many cases may not need treatment. Indication for treatment based on classification and degree of psychosocial impact. In severe acne, therapy should be commenced early to prevent scarring.
Topical preparations:
(1) Benzoyl peroxide; keratolytic agent, encourages skin peeling, and ↓ number of *P. acnes* (S/E: irritation and bleaching of clothes).
(2) Vitamin A derivatives; tretinoin, may take 3–4 months to work.
(3) Azelaic acid.
Antibiotics:
(1) Topical: clindamycin, erythromycin.
(2) Systemic: tetracycline only in >16 years. (S/E: discolours teeth and may soften bones in children.)
A gradual ↑ in *P. acne* resistance to many antibiotics has been documented; growing need to use either appropriate antibiotics or change the therapeutic strategy in favour of other regimens.
Isotretinoin (Roaccutane P.O.): vitamin A derivative, 4–6-month course only by specialist prescription for severe acne (S/E: teratogenic; females require OCP, hyperlipidaemia).
Antiandrogens: in females only; OCP or cyproterone acetate.
UVB: adjunctive therapy, but rarely used.
Advice: improvement may not be seen for at least a couple of months, use non-greasy cosmetics, wash face daily, moderate exposure to sunshine is beneficial.

Acne vulgaris continued

C: **Physical:** facial scarring (atrophic/keloid), hyperpigmentation of scars, 2° infection and fistulae.
Psychosocial: lack of self-confidence.

P: Generally improves spontaneously over months/years. Persists into adulthood in 22% of women and 3% of men.

D: Abnormalities of the female genital tract not present at birth.

A: **Labial adhesions:** adherence of the labia minora in the midline; may give the appearance of absence of the vagina. A thin pale semi-translucent membrane covers the vaginal os. Trauma causes denudation of the epithelial layer of the labia minora mucosa and leads to fibrous tissue formation; therefore sealing of the labia minora. Trauma can involve inflammatory conditions (vulvitis, vulvovaginitis), sexual abuse, or straddle injuries.
Vulvovaginitis: pruritus, vulval pain, vulval erythema, vaginal discharge or bleeding. Usually associated with poor perineal hygeine, constipation, and atopic dermatitis caused by local irritants (bubble bath, soaps, shampoo) or by occlusive clothing causing irritation. May be caused by trauma 2° to abuse; therefore this should be considered if other concerns are present.

A/R: Vulvovaginitis is often misdiagnosed as a UTI due to its similar presentation.

E: **Labial adhesions:** peak age: 3 months to 6 years, incidence: 1–2%.
Vulvovaginitis: very common in < 5-year-olds.

H: **Labial adhesions:** usually asymptomatic and noted on routine examination. Some patients may leak urine when they stand after voiding.
Vulvovaginitis: history should include toilet-training, type of nappy used, bad odour or dark discharge, scratching, history of eczema, allergic rhinitis, or diarrhoea, tendency of child to insert objects, and any possible indication of abuse.

E: **General:** should be by a skilled clinician, in a well-lit room with a relaxed and distracted child (mother reading book).
Labial adhesions: the edges of the labia minora are sealed along the mid-line, beginning at the posterior fourchette and extending anteriorly towards the clitoris.
Vulvovaginitis: commonly, only vulvitis will be detected, although vaginal discharge and bleeding may also be present.

P: See **A**.

I: Exclude other vaginal disorders such as imperforate hymen or septate vagina prior to treatment.
Microbiology: vaginal swab if discharge present, MSU.
Radiology: indirect cystourethrogram may show urinary retention behind the fused labia, bladder distention +/− hydronephrosis in labial adhesions.

M: **Labial adhesions:** oestrogen cream dissolves the adhesions in 90% of cases. Once adhesions have been lysed vasoline is used as prophylaxis for 1–2 months.
Vulvovaginitis:
- Treat any underlying infection with appropriate antibiotics.
- Education of adequate perineal hygiene and removal of potential irritants.

C: **Labial adhesions:** without adequate treatment 20–40% will develop UTI.

P: **Labial adhesions:** recurrence is common, therefore good follow-up is required.
Vulvovaginitis: outcome good with improved perineal hygiene.

CONDITIONS

Anaemia, aplastic

D: Pancytopaenia (deficiency of all blood cell elements) associated with bone marrow aplasia.

A: **Idiopathic (> 40%):** may be mediated by immunological suppression of multipotent myeloid stem cells by cytotoxic T cells.
Acquired:
(1) Viral infection (parvovirus, EBV, CMV, HIV, hepatitis, measles).
(2) Drugs (chloramphenicol, alkylating agents, methotrexate).
(3) Chemicals (DDT, benzene).
(4) Radiation.
(5) PNH
Inherited:
(1) Fanconi anaemia (AR, error of DNA repair).
(2) Congenital dyskeratosis (sex-linked disorder with skin and nail atrophy).
(3) Schwachman Diamond syndrome: AR disorder with pancreatic insufficiency, skeletal abnormalities and recurrent infections. Pancytopaenia in 25%.

A/R: Fanconi anaemia may be associated with growth retardation, abnormalities of forearm bones, heart and renal tract defects (horseshoe or pelvic kidney), and skin pigmentation.

E: **Incidence:** 2–5/1 000 000/year. Can occur at any age. M > F.

H: May present with slow (months) or rapid (days) onset:
(1) ↓**RBC:** tiredness, lethargy, and dyspnoea.
(2) ↓**Platelets:** easy bruising, bleeding gums, epistaxis.
(3) ↓**WCC:** ↑frequency and severity of infections.

E: Pallor, petechiae, bruises, bacterial or fungal infections.
No hepatomegaly, splenomegaly, or lymphadenopathy.

P: **Macro:** pale or white bone marrow.
Micro: hypocellular bone marrow composed of empty marrow spaces, fat cells, fibrous stroma, and isolated foci of lymphocytes and plasma cells. Classic *chicken wire* appearance.

I: **Bloods:** ↓Hb, ↓platelets, ↓neutrophils, normal MCV, low/absent reticulocytes.
Blood film: to exclude leukaemia.
Bone marrow trephine biopsy: for diagnosis and exclusion of other causes (bone marrow infiltration: lymphoma, leukaemia, malignancies).
Chromosomal abnormalities: ↑random breaks in peripheral lymphocytes in Fanconi anaemia.
Ham's test: for PNH; measures sensitivity of affected RBCs to lysis by complement following activation.

M: **Treat the underlying cause:** review medication taken by patient, treat underlying infection.
Supportive: blood and platelet transfusions as needed, antibiotics for infections, consider antibiotic prophylaxis.
Medical: corticosteroids, cyclosporin A, for Fanconi anaemia; androgen (oxymetholone) (S/E: virilisation, liver toxicity).
BMT: definitive treatment; from an HLA-matching sibling in younger patients (< 20 years). Cure rate up to 90%.

C: **Complication of disease process:** bleeding, sepsis and ↑risk of developing myelodysplastic syndromes or leukaemia if the duration of illness is prolonged.
Complication of BMT: graft rejection, GVHD, infection (new or reactivated).

P: Poor prognostic features include:
(1) Platelet $< 10 \times 10^9$/L.
(2) Neutrophil $< 0.5 \times 10^9$/L.
(3) Reticulocytes $< 10 \times 10^9$/L.
➤50% of patients with all these features lasting more than 3 weeks die.

D: Premature erythrocyte breakdown causing decreased (< 120 days) erythrocyte lifespan and anaemia.

A: Intravascular (in the circulation) or extravascular (in the reticuloendothelial system, i.e. broken down by macrophages in the spleen).

A/R: **Hereditary:**

(1) Membrane defects:
- Hereditary spherocytosis: AD condition which leads to abnormal spectrin (a structural membrane protein that alters deformability of RBCs).
- Hereditary elliptocytosis: AD condition.

(2) Red cell enzyme defects:
- G6PD: X-linked disorder which makes RBCs more susceptible to oxidative injury.
- Pyruvate kinase deficiency: AR condition which creates a shift to the right on the oxygen dissociation curve, so patients can tolerate very low Hb.

(3) Haemoglobinopathies: sickle-cell anaemia (see chapters), thalassaemia.

Acquired:

(1) **Immune haemolytic anaemia:**
- **Autoimmune:** warm or cold antibodies attach to RBCs. This leads to activation of complement and subsequent haemolysis of RBCs.
  Warm antibodies: idiopathic/associated with SLE, lymphoma, or drugs (e.g. methyldopa.).
  Cold antibodies: idiopathic/associated with infections (*Mycoplasma*, EBV) or lymphoma.
- **Isoimmune:** transfusion reaction, haemolytic disease of the newborn.

(2) **Non-immune haemolytic anaemia:**
- **Trauma:** RBC fragmentation in abnormal microcirculation; TTP, HUS, DIC, malignant hypertension, pre-eclampsia, artificial heart valves.
- **PNH:** acute onset haemoglobinuria, which is idiopathic or 2° to complement-mediated lysis.
- **Infection:** malaria.

E: **Hereditary causes:** prevalent in African, Mediterranean, and Middle-Eastern populations.
HS: most common inherited haemolytic anaemia in N. Europe.
Age at presentation: depends on aetiology.

H&E: Pallor, jaundice, hepatosplenomegaly, specific signs of underlying pathogenesis.

P: **Blood film (signs of haemolytic anaemia):** leucoerythroblastic picture, microspherocytosis, macrocytosis, nucleated RBCs/reticulocytes, polychromasia.
Blood film (signs of underlying cause): spherocytes, elliptocytes, sickle cells, fragmented RBCs (DIC), malarial parasites, Heinz bodies (G6PD deficiency).
Age at presentation: depends on aetiology.

I: **Bloods:** ↓Hb, ↑MCV due to reticulocytes, ↑unconjugated bilirubin, ↑LDH, ↓haptoglobin, reticulocyte count, blood film.
Urine: ↑urobilirubinogen 2° to excess unconjugated bilirubin, haemoglobinuria.
Direct Coombs' test: identifies RBCs coated with antibodies using antihuman globulin.
Warm antibodies: IgG, agglutinate RBCs at 37°C.
Cold antibodies: IgM, agglutinate RBCs at room temperature.
Hb electrophoresis: Hb variants. (sickle cell, thalassaemia).
Enzyme assays: G6PD deficiency, pyruvate kinase deficiency.
Osmotic fragility test: detects membrane abnormalities (spherocytosis).
Ham's test: PNH.

Bone marrow biopsy (rarely required): erythroid hyperplasia; may be hypoplastic in PNH.

M: **HS:** folate replacement, splenectomy is reserved for severe cases.
HE: most cases asymptomatic.
G6PD: avoid precipitating factors, drugs (aspirin, sulphonamides, co-trimoxazole, nitrofurantoin, chloramphenicol, chloroquine), and fava beans.
Pyruvate kinase deficiency: splenectomy may be beneficial.
Autoimmune: prednisolone, azathioprine/cyclophosphamide, splenectomy.
PNH: blood transfusions (leucocyte-depleted), anticoagulants for thrombotic episodes; BMT is successful in a small number of cases.

C: Renal failure may develop in all cases due to accumulation of RBC breakdown products in the renal tubules.
PNH: can transform into aplastic anaemia or leukaemia.
HS: gallstones, aplastic anaemia in parvovirus infection, megaloblastic and haemolytic crises (↓folate due to hyperactive bone marrow), leg ulcers, and corneal opacities.

P: Depends on the cause.

D: ↓Hb below the reference range for the age and sex of the individual associated with low MCV (< 80 fl) and depleted iron stores.

A: **Nutritional:**
(1) **Exclusive breastfeeding at > 6 months:** at > 6 months breast milk alone is not sufficient to support the extra iron needs related to growth.
(2) **Doorstep cow's milk introduction in the 1st year:** cow's milk has lower bioavailability of iron than breast milk. Formula milk is fortified with 6 mg iron/L.
(3) **Excessive reliance of milk in the 2nd year of life.**
(4) **Behavioural:** food refusal, grazing, dieting, eating disorders.

Blood loss:
Acute: perinatal, postnatal, e.g. peptic ulcer, Meckel's diverticulum.
Chronic:
(1) **GI:** cow's milk protein intolerance, peptic ulcer disease, inflammatory bowel disease, telangiectasia.
(2) **Hookworm:** ancylostoma duodenale in developing countries.
(3) **Menstrual loss.**
(4) **Drug-induced:** use of aspirin in chronic rheumatic disease.

↓Absorption: Crohn's disease, coeliac disease.
↑Demand: preterm infants (↓foetally acquired iron stores), catchup in small for dates infants, after malnutrition, and in adolescence.

A/R: See **A**.

E: **Iron deficiency anaemia is the commonest anaemia worldwide**.
Peak ages: 6 months to 3 years, adolescent girls. Uncommon in infants < 6 months as they have foetally acquired iron reserves (unless preterm).

H: **General:** failure to thrive, ↓exercise tolerance, developmental delay.
Behavioural: anorexia, pica (ingestion of odd materials), irritability, impaired concentration, ↓progress at school.

E: Pallor of skin and mucous membranes, systolic flow murmurs, brittle nails and hair (↓epithelial cell iron), spoon-shaped nails (koilonychia), glossitis (atrophy of tongue papillae), angular stomatitis.

P: **Film:** microcytic, hypochromic (central pallor), anisocytosis (variable sizes), poikilocytosis (variable shapes).

I: **Bloods:** Hb < 10 g/dl after 6 months in a term infant, ↓MCV, reticulocytosis, ↓serum iron, ↑iron-binding capacity, ↓serum ferritin.
Hb electrophoresis: to exclude β-thalassaemia trait.
Bone marrow (only in complicated cases): erythroid hyperplasia and total absence of iron.

M: **Preterm:** fortify breast milk with iron. Use iron-fortified milk formula.
Infants: ↑highly absorbable haem iron sources (meat, fish) and sources of non-haem iron (such as grains) in vegetarian families. Enhance non-haem iron absorption by eating vitamin C–rich foods at the same meal.
Oral ferrous sulphate: maximum rise of Hb 0.25–0.4 g/dl/day.
Blood transfusion: only if child is very anaemic due to risk of cardiac failure.

C: Impaired mental and psychomotor development. High-output cardiac failure in severe cases.

P: Outcome is good if due to ↑demand or nutrition and prompt action is taken. If there is a GI cause of blood loss or malabsorption, outcome is dependent on identification and appropriate treatment of the condition.

Anaemia of prematurity

D: Normocytic, normochromic, hyporegenerative anaemia in a preterm infant associated with a low serum EPO level. Normal Hb levels at birth are 15–25 g/dl; if Hb falls to < 10 g/dl, the infant is considered to be anaemic.

A: (1) **Inadequate RBC production due to low EPO production:** initially the foetal liver produces EPO, during gestation production gradually shifts to the kidneys. The degree of anaemia and hypoxia required to stimulate EPO production is far higher for the foetal liver than for the foetal kidney. As a result, new RBC production in the preterm infant, whose liver remains the major site for EPO production, is blunted despite what may be marked anaemia.
(2) **Shortened foetal RBC lifespan:** foetal RBC has 50–66% of the lifespan of an adult RBC. This is due to ↓intracellular ATP, carnitine, and enzyme activity, and ↑susceptibility to lipid peroxidation and fragmentation. At birth foetal Hb represents 60–90% of Hb. Levels decline to adult levels of less than 5% by 3–6 months of age.
(3) **Blood loss:** during delivery, repeated blood sampling.
(4) **Low iron stores.**
Rarer pathological causes of anaemia in preterm infants:
(1) **Haemolysis:** 2° to ABO/Rh blood group incompatibility or haemoglobinopathies.
(2) **Bone marrow suppression:** 2° to infection or renal failure.
(3) **Bone marrow failure:** aplastic anaemia or malignancy.

A/R: Low birth weight, family history.

E: Frequency is related to the gestational age and birth weight. Up to 80% of low-birth weight (< 2.5 kg) and 95% of extremely low-birth weight (< 1.25 kg) infants require transfusions.

H&E: **Symptoms and signs of anaemia in a preterm infant:**
(1) ↓Activity, which is improved by transfusion.
(2) Poor weight gain despite adequate calorie intake.
(3) Tachypnoea, tachycardia, pallor, and flow murmurs.
(4) If severe, will result in respiratory depression; and episodes of apnoea.

P: See **A**.

I: **Bloods:** Hb < 10 g/dl, normochromic, normocytic; normal Plt and WCC.
Blood film: ↓reticulocyte count (2° ↓EPO), abnormal RBC forms (sickle cells, target cells in thalassaemia), RBC fragmentation (haemolysis).
Blood typing: ABO/Rh blood group incompatibility of neonate and mother.

M: **Indications for packed RBC transfusion:**
(1) Hb < 8 g/dl.
(2) Failure to thrive.
(3) Cardiovascular/respiratory compromise.
(4) Coexisting pathologies that may be exacerbated by anaemia.
Iron supplementation: may reduce need for transfusion.
Recombinant EPO: an alternative when transfusions are not possible due to religious/cultural beliefs. There is conflicting evidence as to whether EPO ↓ the need for transfusions.

C: Transfusion-acquired infection, transfusion-associated fluid overload, electrolyte imbalances, or haemolysis.

P: Preterm infants are usually started on iron therapy for 2–3 months. Anaemia usually resolves spontaneously by 3–6 months, as adult Hb is produced and there is ↑intrinsic RBC and EPO production.

D: Acute inflammation of the appendix.

A: Obstruction of the lumen by impacted faeces → mucosal inflammation. Inflammation then extends into the submucosa to involve the muscular and serosal layers. Fibrinopurulent exudates from the serosal surface extend to the peritoneal surface causing localised peritonitis. The lumen subsequently becomes distended with pus and thrombosis of end-arteries may → gangrene and perforation.

A/R: Poor dietary fibre intake.

E: Commonest cause of an acute abdomen in children.
Prevalence: 4/1000 children.
Can occur at any age, most common > 5 years of age and rare in < 2 years.

H: **There is large variation in clinical picture:**
- Colicky pain starts periumbilically then moves to the RIF and becomes more constant once the peritoneum becomes inflamed. Pain is aggravated by movement.
- Anorexia (beware of child with vague abdominal pain who will not eat favourite food).
- Vomiting in young children.
- Constipation or diarrhoea (less common).
- Low-grade fever.

E: **General:** tachycardia, fever, reluctance to move.
Abdominal: if child is anxious, use their hand to press on belly:
- Rebound/percussion tenderness signifies inflammation of the peritoneum.
- Guarding in RIF (McBurney's point).
- Rovsing's sign (pain more in RIF than in LIF when the LIF is pressed).

Rectal: should be performed by the most senior doctor where indicated. There is marked tenderness against anterior rectal wall, especially with a retrocaecal appendix.

P: See **A**.

I: **Do not delay surgery for investigations.**
Bloods: ↑WCC (normal WCC does not exclude appendicitis), ↑CRP, U&E (especially if vomiting).
Urine: microscopy and culture to exclude UTI.
AXR: may show dilated loops of bowel and a fluid level in the RIF.
USS: may show appendix mass/abscess.

M: **Conservative:** monitor overnight if signs and investigations are equivocal but symptoms are suggestive of appendicitis. Re-examine often.
Surgical: open or laparoscopic appendicectomy with pre-op IV cefuroxime and metronidazole to reduce wound infection.
Appendix mass: inflamed appendix surrounded by omentum:
- **Conservative:** IV cefuroxime and metronidazole, keep NBM. If the mass resolves, do an interval (delayed) appendicectomy.
- **Surgery:** if appendix mass enlarges/patient becomes more toxic (↑pain, ↑temperature, ↑pulse, ↑WCC).

Perforation: fluid resuscitation, correction of electrolytes, and broad-spectrum antibiotics. Usually requires appendicectomy.

C: Perforation, peritonitis (may → adhesions and bowel obstruction or infertility later in girls).

P: Good with skilled surgery. Peritonitis may cause severe illness requiring weeks for full recovery.

Asthma

D: Chronic inflammatory airways disease characterised by variable reversible airway obstruction, airway hyper-responsiveness, and bronchial inflammation.

A: **Genetic factors:** positive family history of asthma or atopy; tendency of T lymphocytes to drive production of IgE on exposure to allergen.
Environmental triggers: passive or active smoking, URTIs, exercise, cold weather, allergens (rare); house dust-mites, pets, seasonal.

A/R: Eczema, allergic rhinitis, family history of atopy, previous CLD of prematurity, previous hyper-reactivity, preterm infants, 'hygiene' hypothesis (exposure to microbial products in infancy aids in switching off mast cell hyper-reactivity).
DD in < 2 years: aspiration, pneumonia, bronchiolitis, tracheomalacia, CF.

E: **Prevalence:** 5–10%. **Age:** 80% of children are symptomatic by the age of 5. M : F = 2 : 1; equalises in adulthood. **Distribution:** viral-associated wheeze/recurrent wheezy bronchitis is ↑ in urban areas and in children of low-socio-economic status families.

H: **Age-related symptoms:**
< 1 year: persistent or recurrent nocturnal cough, wheezing with URTIs.
2–3 years: nocturnal cough, wheezing during exercise with URTIs.
< 5 years: non-productive cough may be the only symptom, often worse at night and in the morning.
Assess severity: frequency of attacks (mild: < 1 attack in 2 months; moderate: > 1 attack in 2 months; severe: persistent symptoms, ↓exercise tolerance), effect on school attendance, hospital attendances, and admissions to PICU.

E: **Respiratory:** end expiratory wheeze, recession, use of accessory muscles, tachypnoea, hyper-resonant percussion note, diminished air entry, hyperexpansion, Harrison's sulcus (anterolateral depression of thorax at insertion of diaphragm).
Peak flow: useful in > 5 years of age; use as baseline (predicted best) and as determinant for efficacy of treatment.
***BTS Guidelines* for assessment of acute asthma attack:**

Severe asthma:
(1) Too breathless to speak or feed.
(2) Tachycardia:
- > 120 bpm in 2–5 years.
- > 130 bpm in < 2 years.

(3) Tachypnoea:
- > 30 breaths/min in 2–5 years.
- > 50 breaths/min in < 2 years.

(4) Peak flow:
- < 50% predicted in > 5 years.

Life-threatening asthma:
(1) Silent chest.
(2) Cyanosis.
(3) Poor respiratory effort.
(4) Hypotension.
(5) Exhaustion.
(6) Confusion.
(7) Coma.
(8) Peak flow:
- < 33% predicted in > 5 years.

P: **Acute phase (within minutes):** ↑airway receptor hyper-responsiveness → narrowing of airways.
Late phase (onset after 2–4 hs, effect may last up to 3–6 months): persistent bronchoconstriction 2° to vicious cycle of inflammation, oedema and excess mucous production.

I: **Few investigations are required.** In severe cases CXR to exclude pneumothorax.

M: ***BTS Guidelines* for the management of acute asthma attack:**

(1) High-flow oxygen via reservoir bag.
(2) Salbutamol and ipratropium bromide via volumatic spacer or nebulised. Salbutamol can be given IV in severe attack.
(3) Oral prednisolone 20 mg (2–5 years), 30–40 mg (> 5 years) or IV hydrocortisone if unable to retain oral medication.
(4) If not responding (< 92% O_2 saturations) or any life-threatening features present, discuss with PICU for ventilatory support.
(5) Aminophylline infusion.
(6) Magnesium sulphate is not indicated in children at present (conflicting evidence).

Discharge criteria: patients can be discharged when stable on 3–4-hourly inhaled bronchodilators. Peak flow 75% of predicted best, and O_2 saturations > 94%.

Education: on adherence to medication, recognition of acute attacks, emergency protocol, maintaining normal activities.

***BTS* stepwise management of chronic asthma:**

Key principles:

(1) Avoid obvious precipitants, e.g. passive smoking.
(2) Ensure good inhaler technique +/− volumatic spacer.
(3) Check compliance.
(4) Review treatment every 3–6 months.
(5) 'Rescue' prednisolone in acute deterioration.

Children < 5 years:

Step 1: mild intermittent asthma; short-acting β_2-agonist inhalers (e.g. salbutamol) as necessary. If used > 1/day → Step 2. Oral salbutamol is useful in children who have difficulties using inhalers +/− volumatic spacers.

Step 2: regular preventor control; add low-dose inhaled steroid (e.g. fluticasone) or leucotriene inhibitor if steroid cannot be used.

Step 3: add-on therapy; trial of leucotriene inhibitors.

Step 4: persistent poor control: refer to respiratory paediatrician.

Children 5–12 years:

Step 1: mild intermittent asthma; short-acting β_2-agonist inhalers as necessary. If used > 1/day → Step 2.

Step 2: regular preventor control; add low-dose inhaled steroid or nedocromil sodium (benefit in 5–12 years).

Step 3: add-on therapy; add LABA e.g. salmeterol.

(1) Good response: continue LABA.
(2) Benefit from LABA but control still inadequate: ↑dose of inhaled steroids.
(3) No response to LABA: stop LABA, ↑dose of inhaled steriods, and add trial of oral theophylline (monitor plasma levels) or leucotriene inhibitor.

Step 4: persistent poor control; further ↑dose of inhaled steroids.

Step 5: continuous or frequent use of oral steroids; maintain ↑dose of inhaled steroids. Add oral prednisolone at lowest dose to provide adequate control. **Refer to respiratory paediatrician**.

C: Growth retardation from disease or treatment with steroids, chest wall deformity, recurrent infections, status asthmaticus can be fatal.

P: Asthma often remits during puberty, and many children are symptom-free as adults, especially those who have mild asthma and are asymptomatic between attacks, or who develop asthma at > 6 years. Rates of admission and mortality in asthma have ↓since the early 1990s.

Atrial septal defect (ASD)/AVSD

D: Congenital defects of the atrial septum, atrioventricular valve and ventricular septum.

A: **Secundum ASD:** defect in centre of atrial septum involving fossa ovalis.
Primum ASD (partial AVSD): defect in lower atrial septum, involving the left atrioventricular valve.
Complete AVSD: large central defect due to ASD and VSD with a single large AV valve.

A/R: All defects are associated with a wide variety of chromosomal and genetic disorders and syndromes. 50% of patients with AVSD have Down syndrome.

E: 4/100 000 live births.

H: Can be asymptomatic or symptomatic depending on the size of the defect. Symptoms for large defects include recurrent respiratory infections, symptoms of CHF, dyspnoea, palpitations (older children) and failure to thrive.
ASD: Acyanotic

E:

- Left-to-right shunt through the ASD once pulmonary vascular resistance falls (approx. 1 week after birth).
- Murmurs are due to ↑flow across valves, not the ASD itself. Flow across pulmonary valves → ejection systolic murmur; across tricuspid valve → mid-diastolic murmur.
- Fixed splitting of the 2nd heart sound occurs due to ↑volume causing prolonged contraction time of the right ventricle. Parasternal lift may occur 2° to RVH.

AVSD:

- May be cyanosed at birth.
- No murmur present at birth; may develop in first few weeks.
- Develop pulmonary hypertension as with large VSDs (loud P2).

CXR: normal at birth, ↑ pulmonary markings and cardiomegaly after 1 month.
ECG: superior axis. Biventricular hypertrophy by 2 months old.

P: In the normal foetal circulation an ASD is required to allow blood to bypass the lungs. It should close at the time of birth.

I: **CXR:** RAH, RVH, prominent PA, and ↑pulmonary vascular markings.
ECG: right axis deviation, 1st degree heart block, right bundle branch block, RAH, and RVH.
Doppler + echo: for diagnostic assessment of size of defect and of CHF. Shows right ventricular volume overload and paradoxical ventricular septal motion.

M: **Supportive management:**
(1) Antibiotic prophylaxis for dental surgery and other minor procedures is important in all septal defects, except secundum ASD.
(2) Medical treatment of associated CHF.
Surgical management: all ASDs are usually closed in order to prevent RVH and arrhythmias in later life.
Ostium secundum: closure ideally at age 3–5 years. Closure can be achieved with a self-expandable 'umbrella' device placed in the defect via cardiac catheterisation in 30%. 70% require surgical closure.
Ostium primum: closure ideally at age 3–5 years. 100% surgical closure due to need to repair valve.
Complete AVSD: usually requires correction in infancy to avoid pulmonary vascular damage. May require treatment of ↑ pulmonary vascular resistance at birth if blue.

C: Infective endocarditis, CHF, atrial fibrillation.

P: 95% remain open 5% close spontaneously. Small to moderate defects do not influence lifespan, where as large defects cause significant morbidity and mortality.
AVSD: without correction, children develop Eisenmenger syndrome and severe CHF.

ASD:

P: 95% remain open, 5% close spontaneously. Small to moderate defects do not influence lifespan, whereas large defects cause significant morbidity and mortality.

AVSD:

Without correction, children develop Eisenmenger syndrome and severe CHF.

D: Disorder characterised by attention deficit, hyperactivity, and impulsiveness.

A: **Genetic factors:** twin studies 81–67% concordance; 1st degree relatives have 50% concordance.

Environmental factors: intrauterine complications, maternal smoking, alcohol and drug abuse during pregnancy. Previously linked to children consuming refined sugar or food additives. However, studies have shown that only 5% of children benefited from restricted diet.

A/R: Depression, anxiety, addictive, obsessional, and behavioural disorders, learning difficulties including receptive and expressive language problems.

E: 3–5% school-age children affected (DSM-IV). M : F = 4 : 1. Onset usually <7 years, symptoms last >6 months.

H&E: **Attention deficit:** inability to sustain mental effort, listen, organise, or finish tasks.

Hyperactivity: fidgeting, running, climbing, or talking excessively.

Impulsiveness: inability to wait their turn, intruding, or interrupting others.

Typically present with disruptive or disobedient behaviour at nursery school.

P: **PET scan studies:** show lower level of activity in the brain areas that control attention. The suggested abnormality is of ascending projections of catecholaminergic and serotonergic neurons into the frontal cortex.

I: ADHD may coexist and/or mimic a variety of developmental, psychological, learning, and language difficulties. Therefore it is important to evaluate each child comprehensively and take a full developmental, educational, and behavioural history. Exclude medical conditions such as impaired vision and hearing or, less commonly, epilepsy (absence seizures) or hypothyroidism.

M: **Mental health professional:**

- Behaviour modification programmes for the home, school, and workplace.
- Parental positive reinforcement of desired behaviour and appropriate negative feedback for unacceptable behaviour.
- Training in social skills and psychotherapy to improve self-esteem.

1st line treatment:

Methylphenidate (Ritalin):

- Psychostimulant which increases arousal in areas of inactivation, thereby improving attention span and reducing impulsivity and hyperactivity.
- S/E: exacerbation of tics; should not be used in children with tics.
- S/E: weight/growth retardation and hypertension; should be monitored every 6 months.

2nd line treatment:

Tricyclic antidepressants:

- Used in patients who do not respond to stimulants or have significant side-effects (tics, severe loss of appetite, marked insomnia).
- Useful in coexisting depression.

Clonidine (α-agonist):

- Useful in children with comorbid tics.
- Use with caution (S/E: agranulocytosis).

C: ADHD often negatively affects a person's educational achievements. This can contribute to economic, social, and life adjustment problems throughout a person's life.

P: Hyperactivity symptoms may improve with maturation and development of self-control. However, adults may suffer from a high turnover of jobs and relationships due to a low level of frustration. Patients who have appropriate educational input, enough support, and good compliance to treatment have the best prognosis.

D: Pervasive developmental disorder mainly affecting communication and social function. Autism is referred to as a 'spectrum disorder', which means that the symptoms and characteristics may vary in their severity of presentation.
(1) **Childhood autism:** severe classical autism.
(2) **Atypical autism:** spectrum of pervasive developmental disorder.
(3) **Asperger's syndrome:** social impairment with preservation of language development.

A: Genetic factors; concordance is 80% in monozygotic twins.
Maternal rubella infection is associated with higher rates of autism.
A link with the MMR vaccine has not been substantiated.

A/R: TS, fragile-X syndrome. Epilepsy may be present in 25%.

E: **There is a wide range of estimates for UK incidence:**
(1) Childhood autism: 3–9/1000 live births; M : F = 4 : 1. Onset < 3 years.
(2) Atypical autism: 1/1000 live births; M : F = 4 : 1.
(3) Asperger's syndrome: 3/1000 live births; M : F = 10 : 1.

H&E: **Motor:** stereotypical and repetitive motor mannerisms (hand-flapping, waving fingers in front of eyes), clumsy and uncoordinated movements.
Behavioural: ritualistic behaviour, the disruption of which → violent temper tantrums. May develop an obsessive interest in one topic (train schedules or toothbrushes) that is odd in its intensity and excludes most other activities.
Social: indifference to others, avoiding eye contact and preferring to be alone, limited gestures and facial expressions, limited understanding of others' gestures, lack of understanding of social rules, attachments to unusual objects.
Speech: delayed speech and language development (not Asperger's), echolalia and poor comprehension, abnormal vocal intonation, hoarse, high-pitched, or monotone.
Learning disability: common and varies with severity of autistic spectrum.
Sensory: may have varying levels of sensitivity to light, touch and sound stimuli.

P: **Abnormal social interaction:** 'Normal children learn social habits without being consciously aware of them. It is these instinctive relations that are disturbed in autistic children. They have to learn everything via the intellect.' (Hans Asperger)

I: **MRI/CT brain:** may show abnormalities in the cerebellum, frontal lobe, and temporal lobe.
Others: IQ testing, EEG (if presenting with fits/funny turns).

M: **Multidisciplinary approach:** behavioural, psychological, and educational interventions should be initiated as early as possible. Children at the severe end of the autistic spectrum disorder may require special school attendance. Support for parents to deal with a severely limiting handicap.

C: **Physical:** abuse from frustrated parents or annoyed social contacts.
Psychological: may result in aggressive or self-injurious behaviour.

P: Varies with degree of severity of autistic spectrum, as this also determines IQ and degree of speech development. Adults with severe autism usually live with their parents or require care in special communities. At the milder end of the spectrum many can attend higher education, be employed successfully and lead independent lives.

D: A developmental condition in which the child experiences a brief episode of silent expiration followed by apnoea.

A: **Pallid (or white) breath-holding attacks:** abnormally sensitive response to carotid sinus or ocular compression with the production of temporary asystole or marked bradycardia.

Cyanotic (or blue) breath-holding attacks: mechanism unclear; however, includes centrally mediated reduced respiratory effort and altered lung mechanics, which may inappropriately stimulate pulmonary reflexes, thus resulting in apnoea and hypoxia.

A/R: 25% of children have a positive family history of breath-holding attacks.

E: Occurs in 1–2% of children between the ages of 6 months and 5 years, 75% of which occur between 6 and 18 months. M = F. Breath-holding spells usually occur from 1–2×/day to 1–2×/month. 60% have cyanotic type, 20% pallid type, and 20% a combination.

H:

Pallid breath-holding attack

Triggered by fear or a painful stimulus such as a knock to the head or falling

↓

Child stops breathing and rapidly loses consciousness

↓

Child becomes pale and hypotonic

↓

May experience a tonic seizure as a result of cerebral underperfusion (reflex anoxic seizure)

Cyanotic breath-holding attack

Triggered by anger, frustration, upsetting event, or scolding

↓

Child cries and subsequently holds breath in expiration

↓

Rapid onset of cyanosis that may progress to loss of consciousness

↓

Brief tonic-clonic jerks, opisthotonos (rigidity and arching of the back, with head thrown backwards)

↓

Bradycardia may follow

Attacks last less than a minute. There is usually full resumption of normal activity within minutes. Some children may remain lethargic and drowsy for some time after an attack.

E: Neurological examination to exclude focal signs suggestive of an underlying structural abnormality such as a myelomeningocele.

P: Involuntary reflex response to a shock, which causes overactivity of the autonomic nervous system that controls breathing and HR.

I: **EEG:** shows generalised slow waves with flattening during the attack (a pattern characteristic of cerebral hypoxia). *Interictally* the EEG is normal.

ECG: if cardiac arrhythmia is suspected.

M: **Parental education:** reassurance and emphasis on consistency and not reinforcing the child's behaviour pattern after the attack. Child should lie flat during attack to ↑cerebral perfusion. Atropine sulphate may be considered in refractory pallid attacks to block the vagus nerve.

C: No immediate complications except if the child collapses in an unsafe environment.

P: Children usually stop having the attacks after the age of 5 or 6 years. Children who have pallid attacks have an ↑incidence of syncope in adulthood. There is no ↑incidence of epilepsy in either type.

Bronchiolitis, acute

D: LRTI characterised by coryza followed by persistent cough, breathlessness, hyperinflation of the chest, and expiratory wheeze in infants <1 year old.

A: RSV in 75%, but there may be multiple causative agents such as rhinovirus and occasionally parainfluenza, influenza, and adenovirus.

A/R: More common and severe in infants with CLD of prematurity, CHD, CF, and immunodeficiency. Breastfeeding and parental avoidance of smoking are protective.

E: Commonest LRTI in infants <1 year old. Winter epidemics: 1–2% infants admitted to hospital.

H: Persistent cough, breathlessness, and expiratory wheeze. In more severe cases infants may become too breathless to feed, have apnoeic spells or become lethargic.

E: **General:** mild pyrexia, tachycardia.
Signs of respiratory distress: tachypnoea, subcostal/intercostal recession, nasal flaring, and widespread expiratory wheeze +/− fine end-inspiratory crackles.
Signs in severe disease: cyanosis, ↓GCS.

P: **Micro:** inflammation of the bronchioles with secretion of mucous, necrosis of ciliated epithelium, and oedema of the submucosa causing airway obstruction.

I: **Bloods:** ↑WCC, ↓Na (2° to SIADH), capillary gas (↓pO_2 and ↑pCO_2 if child is becoming exhausted).
CXR: shows hyperinflation due to small airways obstruction and air trapping. Collapse and/or consolidation may be seen occasionally.
Serology: RSV may be identified by immunofluorescent staining of nasopharyngeal secretions using specific viral antisera.

M: **Criteria for admission:** feeding difficulty, RR >50, episodes of apnoea.
Supportive management: O_2 via nasal cannula or headbox to keep saturations $>96\%$, feeding via NG tube, adequate fluid intake with IV support if necessary.
Active treatment: bronchodilators are of unproven benefit. Steroids are rarely indicated. High-risk infants: may be given antivirals (ribavirin) via SPAG. Ribavirin is teratogenic, therefore care must be taken not to expose mothers/staff who are pregnant.
Criteria for ventilation (5%): signs of exhaustion, recurrent prolonged apnoeas, signs of cerebral hypoxia; drowsy/unrousable.
Prevention: high-risk infants (CLD of prematurity, CHD, CF, immunodeficiency) are given monthly RSV monoclonal antibody prophylaxis (Palivizumab) over the winter period.

C: 1% progress to respiratory failure. Cardiac failure may occur, predominantly in children with an underlying cardiac condition. Acute bronchiolitis does not ↑predisposition towards asthma.

P: Most recover uneventfully in 7–10 days. Wheeze recurs in 50–75% of infants. Diarrhoea can complicate the recovery phase. Mortality is generally very low, but is higher in infants <6 months or with underlying chronic conditions. Mortality rises to 33% if ventilation is required.

D: Bleeds inside the extradural, subdural, or subarachnoid space.

A: **Extradural:** direct head trauma causing arterial or venous bleeding.
Subdural: birth trauma, forceps delivery, low–birth weight infants, high falls, and NAI caused by shaking.
Subarachnoid: ruptured berry aneurysm or arteriovenous malformation.

A/R: May be exacerbated by coagulopathy.

E: **Extradural:** in children 50% occur <2 years. M : F = 4 : 1.
Subdural: occur mainly in young infants. **Subarachnoid:** rare in children.

H&E: All intracranial haemorrhage may develop symptoms and signs of raised ICP as in all cases there is accumulation of blood within a closed cavity:
Early signs ↑ICP: nausea, vomiting, confusion, drowsiness.
Late signs ↑ICP: Cushing response (↑BP, ↓HR), ipsilateral 3rd nerve palsy papilloedema, coma.
Extradural: history of trauma, force and site of impact, severe headache, boggy haematoma.
Acute subdural: shock, seizures and coma, retinal haemorrhages.
Chronic subdural: macrocephaly, failure to thrive, developmental delay.
Subarachnoid: sudden onset occipital headache, retinal haemorrhages, neck stiffness, fever, seizures, and progression to coma.

P: **Extradural:** trauma affecting the middle meningeal artery over the temporal bone.
Subdural: tearing of the veins between the arachnoid and pia mater can give rise to chronic subdural. Acute subdural may occur in neonates by rupture of the vein of Galen.
Subarachnoid: saccular or berry aneurysms arise because of haemodynamic stress in intracranial arteries that are susceptible (e.g. Ehlers–Danlos syndrome, Marfan syndrome).

I: **Bloods:** Hb, clotting screen.
Skull X-ray: may show fracture particularly over temporal bone region.
CT: best modality for detecting blood in the extradural/subdural space or CSF.
Lumbar puncture: xanthochromia (subarachnoid).
Angiography: may show aneurysms or AV malformations in subarachnoid haemorrhage.

M: **Supportive care:** ventilatory support and blood transfusions if shocked.
Treatment of ↑ICP: diuretics (mannitol) and hyperventilation.
Extradural: surgical evacuation of haematoma and coagulation of bleeding sites. Burr holes into the side of the dilated pupil if no neurosurgical consultation is available and if patient is in rapid deterioration with impending herniation.
Subdural: surgical evacuation of haematoma.
Subarachnoid: surgical correction of AV malformation or radiological clipping of aneurysm.

C: Hydrocephalus, uncal/central herniation 2° to ↑ICP, cerebral ischaemia, vasospasm and re-bleeds in subarachnoid haemorrhages.

P: **Extradural:** good with early intervention, GCS prior to surgery correlates well with mortality and neurological sequelae.
Chronic subdural: depends on the cause and associated brain injury. 3% mortality rate. At follow-up 75% have normal development.
Acute subdural: $>60\%$ mortality.
Subarachnoid: $>60\%$ mortality.

Cerebral palsy

D: Non-progressive disorder of movement and posture.

A: **Antenatal (80%):** cerebral dysgenesis/malformation, congenital infections (rubella, toxoplasmosis, CMV).
Perinatal (10%): hypoxic ischaemic encephalopathy, birth trauma.
Postnatal (10%): meningitis, encephalitis, extradural haemorrhage, IVH, head injury, NAI, hyperbilirubinaemia (kernicterus), prolonged hypoglycaemia.

A/R: **Associated:** epilepsy, learning difficulties, visual impairment, squints, hearing loss, and behavioural disorders.
Risk factors: preterm delivery, low birth weight.

E: 2/1000 live births. Usually presents in infancy.

H&E: **General:** delayed milestones, poor feeding, abnormalities of tone, posture, gait, difficulties with language, and impaired social skills.
Clinical types:
Spastic (70%): affected limbs show ↑tone (clasp-knife), brisk reflexes, and extensor plantar responses:

- **Hemiplegia:** unilateral, arm > leg, fisting and early hand preference < 1 year, characteristic posture of abduction of shoulder, flexion at elbow and wrist, pronation of forearm, and extension of fingers.
- **Diplegia:** legs > arms, hypertonicity of hip adductors → leg 'scissoring'.
- **Quadriplegia:** all 4 limbs affected – arms > legs, poor head control, paucity of movement. Abnormal primitive reflexes and fisting in the first few months.

Dyskinetic (10%): normal progress until 6–9 months, followed by progressive dystonia of lower limbs, trunk, and mouth exaggerated by involuntary movements; athetoid (writhing) and choreographic movements (jerking).
Ataxic (10%): hypotonia, ataxia of trunk and limbs, postural imbalance, intention tremor.
Mixed (10%).

P: **Spastic:**

- **Hemiplegia:** damage to middle cerebral artery territory.
- **Diplegia:** IVH, ventricular dilatation, or periventricular lesion.
- **Quadriplegia:** widespread bilateral cerebral lesions.

Dyskinetic: abnormality of extrapyramidal pathways (basal ganglia, thalamus).
Ataxic: abnormal development of cerebellum.

I: Hearing and visual assessment, EEG if seizure-prone.

M: **Multidisciplinary approach:**
Physiotherapy: early to maintain full ROM, function, normal development and prevent contractures.
Occupational therapy: splints, crutches, walking frames, wheelchairs.
Speech therapy: including control of drooling (oral training).
Orthopaedic: surgery to correct deformity and improve function.
Neurosurgical intervention: may be considered for reducing muscle spasticity or for disabling dystonic movements.
Medical: baclofen or botulinum toxin injections to relieve spasticity.
Genetic counselling.

C: Aspiration pneumonia, failure to thrive.

P: **Spastic Hemiplegia:** delayed but eventually normal gait.
Spastic Diplegia: characteristic gait (knees flexed, toe-walking, and adducted hips).

Spastic Quadriplegia: poor prognosis related to feeding disability and immobility. Sufferers are often totally dependent and life expectancy is significantly reduced. Usually die from chest infections 2° to muscular weakness and poor chest dynamics 2° to kyphoscoliosis.
Dyskinetic: usually unable to walk independently, quality of life can often be poor.
Ataxic: most children walk (though often delayed) with the aid of crutches.

Child abuse

D: Maltreatment of children via neglect, emotional, physical, or sexual abuse.

A: **Carer-inflicted:** family members, babysitter.

A/R: Drug abuse, lack of support, mental illness, learning difficulties, unemployment, high number of siblings.
Munchausen's syndrome by proxy (fabricated and induced illness): child is used to fulfil the parents' need for attention and medical involvement.

E: Apparent rising incidence; however, this may be due to changing definitions, ↑recognition and documentation.

H: **Neglect:** developmental delay, failure to thrive, poor school/health surveillance attendance.
Emotional: rejection of child, verbal harassment, withdrawal of love, threats, and ridicule.
Physical: also known as NAI. History is inconsistent with injury, is delayed, elusive, or vague. Recurrent or characteristic injuries (see **E**xamination).
Sexual: involvement of children/adolescents in sexual activities they do not understand and are unable to give informed consent to, including rape, exposure, and pornography.

E: **Neglect:** unkempt appearance.
Emotional: withdrawn child, lack of eye contact, lack of interaction.
Physical:
(1) Bruises at unusual sites; angle of jaw, fingertip marks on trunk/inner thigh/upper arms from gripping; bruising with outlines of objects used (e.g. belt), slap marks over face or buttocks.
(2) Severe head injury after a fall <1.2 m, retinal haemorrhages (shaking).
(3) Burns and scalds (symmetrical, affecting the back, cigarette burns).
(4) Spiral fractures of the long bones, metaphyseal (ends of long bone) fractures, multiple rib fractures at different stages of healing, and skull fractures (especially <1 yr).
(5) Hair avulsion, torn frenulum.
Sexual: bruising, tears, and abrasions around or on genitalia, reflex anal dilatation, sexually transmitted infection, early teenage pregnancy.

P: 10% of abusers have been abused, 90% (the majority) have not.

I: **Measurements:** height, weight, and head circumference; failure to thrive is closely linked with all forms of abuse.
Photograph of injury sustained: consent is not always required from parent.
Bloods: full clotting screen to exclude bleeding disorders.
X-ray: all suspected fractures.
Skeletal survey: may be indicated in a child <3 years to exclude osteogenesis imperfecta (brittle bone disease caused by a genetic defect in collagen).
Psychiatric consultation: if appropriate for the child or carer.

M: **Immediate action:**
(1) Inform senior paediatrician and child health protection team.
(2) Inform social services and/or police child protection team.
(3) Infants may require admission for immediate protection; most school-age children are managed as outpatients.
Subsequent management:
(1) Convene child protection conference involving teachers, paediatrician, GP, social worker and/or NSPCC.
(2) Child may require addition to the Child Protection Register.
(3) Legal enforcement may be required and child may require foster placement if not safe to go back home.

C: Withdrawal, poor school performance and attendance, truancy, sleep disorders, precocious and inappropriate sexual activity, phobias, and failure to thrive.

P: Children who are abused often develop low self-esteem, fearfulness, aggressive behaviour, become substance abusers, and have difficulties establishing relationships in later life.

Chronic lung disease (CLD) of prematurity

D: Previously known as BPD.

Original: dependence on a ventilator after 28 days with characteristic X-ray changes.

Modified: as infants are now being resuscitated at earlier gestation times, the definition has been modified to ventilation requirement at corrected age of term with characteristic X-ray changes.

A: **Multifactorial in pathology:**

(1) Volutrauma and barotrauma due to PPV.

(2) High inspired oxygen concentration ($FiO_2 > 40\%$) as this is toxic to the immature lung.

(3) Activation of inflammatory mediators (by free radicals, barotrauma, and infection).

(4) Inadequate nutritional supplementation.

A/R: Infants with RDS have ↑ risk of CLD.

E: Inversely related to gestation and birth weight. Incidence is increasing due to the survival of very low–birth weight infants.

H&E: Most appropriately managed neonates are asymptomatic whilst ventilated; however, some may have chronic recession, poor weight gain, and increased energy intake. After being weaned off the ventilator, these children may remain O_2 dependent and require O_2 at home. They are susceptible to multiple respiratory problems in childhood.

P: **Theory of oxygen-mediated lung injury:** results from the generation of superoxides, hydrogen peroxide, and oxygen-free radicals, which disrupt membrane lipids.

Histopathology: interstitial oedema, mucosal metaplasia, interstitial fibrosis, overdistended alveoli.

I: **ABG:** compensated respiratory acidosis reflecting chronic high pCO_2.

CXR: characteristic hyperinflation and cystic changes. Used to determine severity, and distinguishes CLD from atelectasis, pneumonia, and air-leak syndromes.

M: Factors that cause CLD such as PPV, oxygen therapy are necessary for survival in preterm infants; therefore management is primarily about minimisation of risk.

Ventilation: oxygen toxicity, barotraumas, and volutrauma can be minimised by strict monitoring and maintenance of pH, pCO_2, and pO_2 within small ranges, depending on age of preterm infants.

Nutritional support: early parenteral nutrition. Maximisation of nutritional intake prevents further lung injury and aids tissue repair.

Prevention:

(1) Surfactant is used in the treatment of RDS.

(2) Use of steroids to prevent CLD is highly controversial as it has been shown to have an adverse effect on neurodevelopmental outcome. Steroids are generally only used in ventilator-dependent neonates who are 'stuck' on the ventilator.

Long-term: home O_2 supported by community children's nurses; 'hospital-at-home' team.

C: Pulmonary hypertension → cor pulmonale, ↑risk of respiratory infections especially RSV pneumonia (palivizumab; monoclonal antibody prophylaxis for RSV is given monthly over the winter period).

P: With advances in perinatal and neonatal care of preterm infants, survival has improved. However, infants with severe CLD are at high risk in the first 2 years of life. By adolescence the main changes remaining are airways obstruction, airway hyperreactivity, and hyperinflation.

D: Congenital malformation, resulting in clefts that involve the lip, hard palate, and soft palate; may be unilateral or bilateral.

A: **Cleft lip:** failure of fusion of the frontonasal and maxillary processes.
Cleft palate: failure of fusion of the palatine processes and nasal septum.

A/R: Family history. Associated with 400 syndromes, e.g. Down syndrome.
May be associated with other congenital midline anomalies.
Suggested link with maternal smoking.

E: 1/1000 live births; commonest congenital malformation.
20% are an isolated cleft lip, 50% are both a cleft lip and palate, and 30% are cleft palate alone.

H: **At birth:** overt clefts of the hard +/− soft palate.
Postnatal:
(1) Feeding difficulties: sucking may be compromised due to loss of an oral seal.
(2) Airway difficulties: tongue may prolapse through the cleft into the nasal cavity.
(3) Nasal reflux of liquid or food: in partial clefts of the soft palate.
(4) Hypernasal speech or nasal emission: may be detected later, especially in submucosal clefts.

E: Cleft palate disorders are screened for as part of the neonatal examination (see Appendix). The palate should be palpated posteriorly to exclude a posterior cleft palate and to detect an indentation of the posterior palate from a submucosal cleft.

P: **Cleft lip:** a narrow opening or gap in the skin of the upper lip, all the way to the base of the nose.
Cleft palate: an absence of the palate between the oral and the nasal cavities. Clefts may extend through soft or hard palate or both.

I: **Antenatal USS:** majority of cleft defects are detected at 18–22 weeks.

M: **Multidisciplinary approach:** plastic surgeons, requires input from ENT and dentists, speech therapists, audiologists, nutritionists, specialist children's nurses and social workers.
Advice: slower feeding, positioning the nipple along the noncleft side and towards the back of the mouth, use of cleft palate feeders, semi-upright positioning and regular monitoring for signs of inadequate feeding or dehydration.
Surgical correction: should occur at <1 year to facilitate normal speech and language development. Various surgical techniques:
(1) 1-stage closure involving closure of both the hard and soft palates at 11 months.
(2) 2-stage closure of the soft palate at 3 months and hard palate at 18 months.
(3) If there is delay in repair due to coexisting problems such as cardiac defects, closure will require a pharyngeal flap.

C: ↑ Susceptibility to URTIs, hearing loss, speech defects, dental problems.

P: Good with early surgical repair, children with large defects may still have defective speech.

Coarctation of the aorta (COA)

D: Narrowing of the lumen of the aorta that produces an obstruction to flow.
Preductal: the narrowing is proximal to the ductus arteriosus.
Postductal: the narrowing is distal to the ductus arteriosus.

A: Failure of normal development of the aortic arch in the 5th and 6th week of gestation.

A/R: Turner syndrome, congenital rubella, VSD, PDA, hypoplastic left heart, interruption of the aortic arch (severe form of coarctation with no connection between the proximal and distal aorta).

E: 1/10 000 live births.

H: **Antenatal:** often diagnosed on antenatal USS.
Neonatal: when the ductus arteriosus closes in the 2nd to 3rd week of life, there is a sudden overflow of blood into the left ventricle, which causes LVF (dyspnoea, lethargy, feeding difficulties and failure to thrive).
Infancy: symptoms depend on the severity of stenosis and the development of collateral circulation:

- Preductal COA usually has good collateral circulation.
- Postductal COA has a variable collateral circulation.

Childhood → adulthood: patients with good collateral circulation may be asymptomatic until childhood, adolescence, or adulthood.

E: Nodding head movements accompanying each heart beat, weak femoral pulse, difference in BP between upper and lower limbs (SBP >20), loud S1 and narrow split S2, usually no murmur.

P: Collateral circulation connects the proximal and the distal aspects of the aorta over time. This develops mainly from the subclavian, scapular, internal thoracic, and intercostal arteries. Low BP and flow exist in the arteries that branch off distal to the constriction. High BP occurs in the arteries that branch off closer to the heart. Therefore a high BP exists in the upper body and arms, and a low BP in the lower body and legs.

I: **CXR:** cardiomegaly with ↑pulmonary vascular markings (LVF), a hypoplastic aortic knob with dilated post-stenotic segment of the aorta.
ECG: LVH in older children.
Doppler echo: diagnostic and demonstrates pressure gradient.

M: If COA is diagnosed antenatally, child should be born in a cardiac centre.
Medical: resuscitate ABC. Commence prostaglandin infusion at birth to keep ductus arteriosus open or to reopen if the child presents when the duct closes. Ventilate early.
Surgery: is performed 24 h later; resection of ductal tissue with end-to-end anastomosis or subclavian artery flap repair. There is a 5–10% incidence of re-coarctation after surgery.
Balloon angioplasty: may be used as an alternative to surgery if coarctation is localised or for re-coarctation following surgery. This procedure, however, also has a risk of re-stenosis.

C: **Hypertension 2° to activated renin–angiotensin system:** may cause aortic dissection/rupture, subarachnoid haemorrhage from ruptured berry aneurysm and CAD.

P: Mortality is high if the child is not diagnosed antenatally and presents when the ductus arteriosus closes. Prognosis is good with early surgical intervention. Surgical mortality is $<1\%$. Follow-up is required to monitor for re-stenosis.

D: A lifelong gluten-induced enteropathy of the proximal small bowel resulting in malabsorption, which remits completely on gluten withdrawal.

A: Permanent sensitivity to the α-gliadin component of the cereal protein gluten. The immunological reaction in the small intestine results in mucosal damage and loss of villi.

A/R: Dermatitis herpetiformis (itchy blisters on elbows, knees, face and buttocks), autoimmune thyroid disease, DM, pernicious anaemia, IgA deficiency. 10% are familial.

E: 1/1000 in the UK, 1/300 in SW Ireland (Galway). Falling incidence is attributed to breastfeeding, later weaning, and later introduction of gluten.
Age of presentation: < 5 years. M = F.

H: **Early childhood:** failure to thrive after weaning (where gluten is the weaning diet), diarrhoea, steatorrhoea, irritability, vomiting and anorexia.
Late childhood: anaemia (iron/folate deficiency) or failure to thrive without GI symptoms.
Adolescence: delayed puberty and short stature.

E: Miserable, pale, hypotonic, aphthous stomatitis, digital clubbing, abdominal distension, 'pot-belly' appearance, buttock wasting.

P: **Macro:** 'subtotal villous atrophy' of the proximal small intestine; mucosa has a smooth flat appearance.
Micro: ↑inflammatory infiltrates of lymphocytes and plasma cells in the lamina propria of the small bowel.

I: **Bloods:** ↓Hb, ↓MCV in iron deficiency, ↑MCV in B_{12}/folate deficiency, ↓Ca^{2+}, ↓albumin.
Serology:
(1) Antiendomysial and antigliadin antibodies (IgA antibody; 95% specific unless patient is IgA deficient (2%)).
(2) Antibody directed against *tissue transglutaminase* is a new highly specific and sensitive marker for coeliac disease.
Stool: faecal fat test for steatorrhoea.
Jejunal biopsy: gold standard for diagnosis.
Classical criteria:
(1) Flattened smooth mucosa with subtotal villous atrophy.
(2) Villi return to normal on gluten-free diet.
(3) Proven relapse on gluten challenge for 3 months (only done in children <2 yrs as screening tests are not as reliable and because it may be a transient gluten intolerance).

M: **Nutritional advice:** strict lifelong gluten-free diet (no wheat, barley, or rye products). Oats are compatible with a gluten-free diet. Vitamin and iron supplements.
Pancreatic enzyme supplementation: facilitates weight gain.

C: **Problems in pregnancy:** may result in foetal loss and congenital abnormalities in women with poorly controlled coeliac disease due to folate, iron and vitamin B_{12} deficiency.
Other: osteoporosis and related fractures, ulcerative jejuno-ileitis, 2° lactose intolerance due to damage of the brush border, intestinal lymphoma, bacterial overgrowth and infertility.

P: Many experience apparent spontaneous remission in adolescence but worsening of symptoms in adult life. When there is a strict adherence to a gluten-free diet, there is a good prognosis.

Congenital adrenal hyperplasia

D: Inherited disorder of adrenal steroid synthesis.

A: Autosomal recessive genetic defect in the steroid synthesis pathway. Results in ↓cortisol and, in some cases, ↓aldosterone synthesis. This results in a 2° rise in pituitary ACTH secretion, which causes enlargement of the adrenal glands and build-up of precursor steroids.
Enzyme defects: 21-hydroxylase deficiency (90%), 11β-hydroxylase deficiency (5%) and 17α-hydroxylase deficiency (5%).

A/R: Consanguinity, family history.

E: **Annual incidence:** 21-hydroxylase deficiency: 1/10 000. 11β-hydroxylase deficiency: 1/100 000. 17α-hydroxylase deficiency: 1/100 000.

H&E: **21-hydroxylase deficiency (↑androgen, ↓aldosterone):**
Acute salt-losing crisis: may occur in up to 70% at 2–3 weeks 2° to ↓aldosterone synthesis → vomiting, sweating, dehydration, hyponatraemia, hyperkalaemia, hypotension, and rapidly ensuing coma.
Female virilisation:
Antenatal: ambiguous genitalia, cliteromegaly, fused labia.
Childhood: acne, hirsutism, accelerated growth and skeletal maturation.
Male precocious puberty: early pubic hair, penile and muscle enlargement, accelerated growth and skeletal maturation.
11β-hydroxylase deficiency (↑11-deoxycorticosterone (mineralocorticoid), ↓androgens): hypertension and hypokalaemia; ↑androgen mediated symptoms and signs as for 21-hydroxylase deficiency.
17α-hydroxylase deficiency (↑11-deoxycorticosterone (mineralocorticoid), ↓androgens): hypertension and hypokalaemia.
Females: failure to develop 2° sexual characteristics at puberty.
Males: ambiguous or female genitalia.

P: **Macro:** enlarged adrenal glands.

I: **Bloods:** 17-hydroxyprogesterone (↑in 21-hydroxylase deficiency and 11β-hydroxylase deficiency), testosterone, ↑basal ACTH, LH, FSH, U&E.
ACTH stimulation test: inappropriately elevated 17-hydroxyprogesterone levels after IM ACTH.
Pelvic USS: to exclude POS.
Karyotyping: to confirm gender of infants with ambiguous genitalia.
Molecular genetic testing: to confirm location of mutation.

M: **Acute salt-losing crisis:** IV normal saline, dextrose, and hydrocortisone, monitor for hypoglycaemia.
Medical:
(1) Glucocorticoid replacement with dexamethasone or hydrocortisone.
(2) 9 α-fludrocortisone in salt-losers; monitor regularly for raised BP (S/E: 9 α-fludrocortisone).
(3) Treatment is monitored by measuring serum levels of 17-hydroxyprogesterone and growth.
Surgical: clitoroplasty if enlarged at 4 years, vaginoplasty at puberty.
Genetic counselling: antenatal screening occurs in the UK; CVS for DNA studies, 17-hydroxyprogesterone is raised in amniotic fluid.
Support: psychological counselling for parents and the child.

C: Infertility. Without treatment child may develop short stature due to premature epiphyseal closure. Side-effects from high-dose steroids.

P: Good if diagnosed early. Undiagnosed infants with 21-hydroxylase deficiency may die from salt-losing crises.

Congenital cytomegalovirus (CMV) infection

D: Congenital abnormality caused by antenatal transmission of CMV from the mother to the foetus.

A: **Maternal CMV infection:** may result from 1° maternal infection or recurrent infection. 1° maternal infection is much more likely to cause symptoms and sequelae in the infant.
Congenital CMV infection: transplacental transmission causes viral angitis or a direct teratogenic effect on the developing foetus.
Perinatally acquired CMV infection: aspiration of cervicovaginal secretions in the birth canal.
Postnatally acquired CMV infection: during breastfeeding, but is benign as the infant is simultaneously actively immunised. Contact with family members or other children.

A/R: Congenital CMV infection resulting from 1° maternal infection is more likely to occur in upper socio-economic groups (NEJM).

E: 3–4/100 live births; commonest congenital infection. 50% of pregnant women are susceptible; of these 1% will have a 1° infection during pregnancy, which will cause infant infection in 40%.

H&E: **1° or recurrent CMV maternal infection:** mothers may not be aware of previous CMV infection as it is usually asymptomatic or mild with fever +/− lymphadenopathy and occasionally a sore throat.
Neonatal presentation: 10% of infants infected are symptomatic at birth. Depending on gestational age at time of maternal infection, the infant will present with a different spectrum of pathology:

- **Early gestation:** IUGR, microcephaly, intracranial calcifications.
- **Late gestation:** jaundice, hepatosplenomegaly, petechiae, thrombocytopenia and pneumonia.

Chorioretinitis: occurs in 10–20% with symptomatic disease.
Sensorineural deafness: occurs in 50% of symptomatic and 15% of asymptomatic infants.

P: CMV is a member of the Herpesviridae family of large DNA viruses.

I: **Antenatal:** amniotic fluid culture at 18 weeks gestation.
Virology: isolation from saliva, tears, urine, CSF in the first 2 weeks.
Serology: serum IgM and IgG is less sensitive and specific.
Radiology: CT head for cerebral calcification, abdominal USS to monitor hepatosplenomegaly.

M: **Antenatal:** TOP may be recommended if there is proven infection.
Multidisciplinary approach: involvement of paediatrics, neurology, ophthalmology, ENT, audiology; screen for other pathologies.
Medical treatment: the use of ganciclovir for the treatment of infants with symptomatic congenital CMV infection is being evaluated.
Follow-up: audiological and developmental follow-up are required to identify and manage disabilities at the earliest possible age.
Prevention: there is currently no vaccine available.

C: Infants with intracranial calcifications are more likely to have cognitive and audiologic deficits later in life.

P: Infants infected with 1° CMV, who are symptomatic at birth, will have significant long-term handicap. 10–15% of infected but initially asymptomatic infants will later develop sensorineural deafness or have learning difficulties.

Congenital hypothyroidism

D: Deficiency of thyroid hormone present at birth.

A: **Developmental defects (90% of cases):** aplasia, hypoplasia with ectopy, hypoplasia without ectopy. May be familial or sporadic.
Maternal transmission: use of antithyroid drugs or radioiodine during pregnancy.
2° and 3° hypothyroidism: pituitary defect (abnormal TSH), hypothalamic defect (TRH deficiency).
Inborn errors of thyroid hormonogenesis: ↓TSH responsiveness, Pendred's syndrome; defective thyroglobulin synthesis and transport.
Thyroid hormone resistance.

A/R: Family history.

E: Relatively common: 1/3500 live births. M : F = 1 : 2.

H: **Neonates:** most newborns are asymptomatic due to the transplacental passage of moderate amounts of maternal T_4 (can produce levels in the foetus 25–50% of normal).
Infants: 1st sign is often prolonged neonatal jaundice. Subsequently may develop other symptoms of hypothyroidism including lethargy, slow feeding, excessive sleeping, little vocalisation, and constipation.

E: **Physical signs:** coarse dry hair, flat nasal bridge, protruding tongue 2° to macroglossia, hypotonia, slowly relaxing reflexes, umbilical hernia, slow pulse, and cardiomegaly.
Development: later global developmental delay, learning disability, delayed puberty, dentition and short stature become apparent.

P: See **A**.

I: **Universal neonatal screening:** Guthrie's test (heelprick at 5–7 days) for TSH level (> 50 μU/L is diagnostic). Infants with 2°/3° hypothyroidism or ↓TSH responsiveness are not detected by this method; therefore clinical vigilance is still required.
Bloods: ↓T_4 (not in thyroid-binding globulin deficiency), ↓/↑TSH (depending on the cause), ↓Hb, unconjugated hyperbilirubinaemia (prolonged neonatal jaundice).
Wrist and hand X-rays: bone age < chronological age. The rough 'bone age' is calculated by analysing the number of ossification centres present in the hand and wrist.
Radioactive technetium scan: to detect developmental defects of the thyroid, such as dysgenesis or ectopia.
Echo: may develop cardiomegaly +/− pericardial effusions.

M: Universal neonatal screening, confirmation, and early treatment avoid serious sequelae.
T_4 replacement: the mainstay of treatment; dosage depends on age.
Regular follow-up:
(1) Monitor TSH, T_4 levels, development, and growth.
(2) Monitor bone age to ensure adequate osseous development; will be delayed with undertreatment.
(3) Patients will require lifelong follow-up to monitor for adequate levels of thyroid hormone.

C: **Iatrogenic:** excessive treatment with T_4 → advancement of bone age and later to reduced adult height as the epiphyses fuse prematurely.

P: Linear growth and skeletal maturation respond dramatically to treatment with T_4. The ultimate intellectual level of the patient is inversely proportional to the age at which the patient's treatment is started.

D: Congenital abnormality caused by antenatal transmission of rubella from the mother to the foetus.

A: **1° maternal infection:** adults are often asymptomatic or present with fever, lymphadenopathy, and maculopapular rash.
Antenatal transmission: transplacental during maternal viraemic phase.
Rate of transmission: inversely related to the gestational age: 1st trimester – 75–90%, 2nd trimester – 35–40%, 3rd trimester – 25–50%.
Risk of congenital malformation: varies with gestational age:
$<$ **8 weeks:** classical triad of rubella infection: deafness, CHD, cataracts.
13–16 weeks: impaired hearing (30%).
$>$ **18 weeks:** minimal risk of congenital malformations but may have chronic infection of the eyes, ears and CNS.
Maternal reinfection: rare but can cause congenital rubella infection and teratogenesis.

A/R: Developing countries, young maternal age.

E: There has been a dramatic drop in the number of congenital rubella births and TOP following introduction of the rubella vaccine:

There is potential for ↑ in the future due to ↓uptake of MMR vaccination.

H: Gestation time of maternal infection, maternal immunisation status.

E: **Antenatal:** may cause spontaneous abortion or stillbirth in the most severe of cases. Infants who survive may be preterm or have IUGR.
Neonatal manifestations:
(1) Lethargy/irritability, failure to thrive.
(2) Cardiovascular: PDA, pulmonary valve stenosis, ASD, VSD.
(3) Ocular: cataracts, chorioretinitis, retinitis pigmentosa.
(4) CNS: hydrocephaly, microcephaly, meningoencephalitis, intracranial calcifications, seizures.
(5) GI: jaundice, hepatosplenomegaly.
(6) Respiratory: pneumonitis.
Sequelae (2 months to $>$ 2 years after birth):
(1) Sensorineuronal deafness.
(2) Neurological: progressive rubella panencephalitis.
(3) Endocrine: GH deficiency, hyper/hypothyroidism, DM.

P: Rubella is an RNA virus in the Togaviridae family. In the foetus the virus causes a vasculitis with resultant tissue necrosis without inflammation or direct viral damage of infected cells.

I: **Virology:** isolation from saliva, tears, urine, and CSF in the first 3 months.
Serology: foetal rubella-specific IgM, persistence of rubella-specific IgG after 8–12 months of age.
ELISA: for detection of specific antigens. **Echo:** cardiac defects.
CXR: pneumonitis or pulmonary oedema 2° to CHF.
CT head: intracranial calcifications and other CNS manifestations.

M: **Antenatal:** TOP is recommended if there is proven infection in 1st trimester.
Multidisciplinary approach: involvement of paediatrics, neurology, cardiology, endocrinology, ophthalmology, ENT, audiology; screen for other pathologies.
Surgical management: repair of cardiac defects, glaucoma, cataracts.

C: Global developmental delay, behavioural problems.

P: Mortality is 10–20% in the 1st year. Due to multiorgan pathology, rubella-infected infants have a poor prognosis with lifelong morbidity.

Constipation

D: A child can be classified as having constipation if one or more of the following are true:
(1) Child passes <1 bowel motion every 3 days.
(2) Stools are hard, dry, and may be small (pellets) or unusually large.
(3) Stools are difficult or painful to pass.

A: **Functional:** 90–95% of cases; due to vicious cycle of retention and pain on defaecation.
Dietary: inadequate fluid intake, malnutrition, high-refined carbohydrate and high-protein diet, or a low-fibre diet.
Organic (rare):
(1) GI anomalies: Hirschsprung disease, anorectal stenotic lesions, anal fissures.
(2) Spinal/neuromuscular disease.
(3) Hypothyroidism.

A/R: Cerebral palsy, delayed passage of meconium, failure to thrive, positive family history.

E: **Extremely common:** accounts for 3–5% outpatient consultations and 35% of gastroenterology consultations. **Peak incidence:** 2–4 years of age.

H: **General:** detailed, including diet and social setting, onset of constipation. Delayed passage of meconium >24 h at birth is characteristic of Hirschsprung's disease.
Assessment of stool frequency: infants have a wide range.
During breastfeeding: range is from 10/day to 1 every 10 days. This large range is because breast milk may be completely absorbed; however, some infants with a gastrocolic reflex will pass a motion every time they are breastfed.
During formula-feeding: range is from 3 to 5/day.
Following infancy: at >1 year, child should have range similar to that expected in adulthood: 3/day to 1 every 3 days.

E: May have abdominal distension. Inspection of the anus and digital rectal examination should be performed to exclude fissures or tears.

P: **Functional constipation:** the child begins to associate pain with defaecation and withholds stools in an attempt to avoid discomfort. With ↑retention, sensory feedback from the bowel is reduced, the rectal wall is stretched and loses contractile strength, and water absorption from faecal matter ↑, resulting in larger and harder stool.

I: **Radiology:** AXR may be helpful in the initial assessment.
Anorectal manometry: useful in special cases for discriminating between constipation and Hirschsprung disease.

M: **Stage 1:** dietary changes (↑fibre; fruits, vegetables), adequate fluids, exercise, and regular toileting.
Stage 2: use of laxatives/faecal softeners.
Stage 3: rarely child requires admission to achieve bowel emptying with enemas or bowel-preparing agents.
Specific treatment: lignocaine gel for anal fissures, corrective surgery in Hirschsprung disease.

C: Chronic constipation can result in faecal overload, overflow incontinence, encopresis, and 2° emotional and behavioural difficulties.

P: Only 50% recover within 1 year and 65–70% recover within 2 years; the remainder require laxatives for daily bowel movements or continue to soil for years.

Cow's milk intolerance

D: Transient intolerance to lactose and/or protein found in cow's milk following an infective episode of diarrhoea (usually rotavirus).

A: **Carbohydrate intolerance:** lactose intolerance 2° to mucosal damage to the intestine.
Protein intolerance: immunomediated reaction to cow's milk protein following damage to intestinal mucosa.

A/R: Atopy, adverse reactions to other foods.

E: Widely overdiagnosed; incidence ranges from 0.6% to 7.5% according to different diagnostic criteria and clinical features.

H& E: Preceding infective episode of diarrhoea.
General: irritability, poor feeding, failure to thrive.
Allergic symptoms: nasal discharge, wheeze, eczema, rhinitis.
GI: GORD, vomiting, colic, persistent diarrhoea that may have intermittent frothy explosive stools 2° to lactose intolerance.

P: **Lactose intolerance:** disaccharide enzymes (for lactose, sucrose, and maltose) are located at the brush border of the absorptive cells. Mucosal damage reduces the activity of these enzymes.
Immunomediated protein intolerance: mucosal damage may result in abnormal sensitisation to dietary antigens.

I: **Bloods:** IgE RAST testing is not very sensitive or specific.
Markers of malabsorption: ↓Hb, normocytic or ↓MCV, ferritin, iron, folic acid, albumin.
Stool sample: for MC+S and in lactose intolerance stools are acidic and contain undigested sugar.
Jejunal biopsies: rarely needed to differentiate from coeliac disease.
Gold standard: symptom resolution once cow's milk has been eliminated from the diet. The diagnosis is then confirmed with at least one positive challenge, performed as an inpatient in case of anaphylaxis, preferably on a double-blind basis.

M: **Prevention:** encourage breastfeeding in all women for a minimum of 6 months (WHO guidelines) to prevent introduction of cow's milk until later and for its other numerous benefits (see appendix).
Carbohydrate intolerance: lactose-free milk for 4–6 weeks to allow mucosal regeneration.
Protein intolerance: alternatives to cow's milk:

(1) **Soya milk formulae:**
  - 50% of cow's milk protein–sensitive infants are also sensitive to soya milk protein.
  - Rich source of phytoestrogens. Controversial as to whether beneficial (protect against breast and prostate cancer) or harmful (infertility, liver disease).

(2) **Goat's milk:** deficient in vitamins and contains no folate.

(3) **Protein hydrolysate formulae:**
  - *Whey-based hydrolysate formulae* – whey in the cow's milk protein is broken down, making it less allergenic than the whole protein in regular formulae.
  - *Casein hydrolysate formulae* – contains smaller protein fragments and amino acids.

(4) **Amino acid–based infant formulae:** contain protein in its simplest form, recommended if condition does not improve with a switch to one of the hydrolysate formulae above.

Gradual reintroduction of cow's milk after 1 year.

C: Malabsorption, failure to thrive, anaphylaxis.

P: Cow's milk intolerance is usually transient and most children tolerate milk products by age 2 years.

D: Hypersensitivity reaction to protein in cow's milk used to make standard baby formula feeds.

A: **Cow's milk protein:** β-lactoglobulin (main cause), α-lactoglobulin, casein, bovine serum albumin, γ-lactoglobulin.

A/R: Family history of atopy.

E: **UK figures:** 4.4% of children aged 1 year, 1.9% aged 2 years, and 0.4 % aged 4 years (Isle of Wight 1997). Condition is much overdiagnosed depending on different diagnostic criteria and clinical features.

H&E: Symptoms appear within the 1st week of introducing cow's milk protein into the infant's diet.
Acute severe reaction: may present with some or all of the following signs of an allergic reaction culminating in acute anaphylaxis:
(1) **Skin:** itch, urticaria, and angio-oedema.
(2) **Respiratory:** wheeze 2° to bronchospasm, stridor 2° to laryngeal oedema.
(3) **Cardiovascular:** tachycardia, hypotension.
(4) **GI:** vomiting, diarrhoea, abdominal pain.
Delayed reaction: eczema, wheeze, and diarrhoea may recur 12–24 h after initial reaction.

P: **Acute reaction:** exposure to allergen in a presensitised individual results in cross-linking of IgE. This triggers mast cell degranulation releasing histamine and leucotrienes in the skin, lungs, gut, and systemically.
Delayed reaction: T-cell mediated; may be caused by cow's milk protein binding to the immature gut and subsequent sensitisation.

I: **Bloods:** ↑IgE, eosinophilia.
Skinprick test: positive in 25% to milk protein.
Gold standard: symptom resolution once cow's milk has been eliminated from the diet. Diagnosis is confirmed with at least one positive challenge, performed as an inpatient, preferably double-blind.

M: **Acute management of anaphylaxis:** weight (kg) = 2(age in years + 4).
(1) Adrenaline IM10 μg/kg = 0.1 ml/kg of 1 : 10 000; may require repeated doses every 15 min until stabilised.
(2) Oxygen +/− ventilatory support if necessary.
(3) Chlorpheniramine 0.2 mg/kg IV.
(4) Hydrocortisone 4 mg/kg IV.
(5) IV resuscitation if shocked (20 ml/kg colloid).
(6) Nebulised salbutamol if wheeze present.
Cow's milk protein alternatives (see **Cow's milk intolerance**).
Prevention: encourage breastfeeding in all women for a minimum of 6 months (WHO guidelines) to prevent introduction of milk protein until later and for its other numerous benefits (see appendix).
Gradual reintroduction of cow's milk after 1 year: if child still shows symptoms of cow's milk protein allergy, 'challenges' with cow's milk may be repeated every 3–6 months as an inpatient in case of anaphylaxis.

C: Anaphylaxis is a real and severe complication of cow's milk protein allergy and can be fatal.

P: 30% of affected individuals tolerate milk by the age of 2 years, although 20% may take >6 years. These children have ↑risk of allergic rhinitis, asthma, eczema, and other food allergies.

Croup (acute laryngotracheobronchitis)

D: Common condition characterised by progressive spread of inflammation down the respiratory tract starting at the larynx, followed by trachea and bronchi 2° to a viral infection.

A: Parainfluenza virus is the most common cause, but other viruses can produce a similar picture, such as RSV, influenza, rhinoviruses.

A/R: **DD of acute stridor:** acute epiglottitis (child is toxic, no cough, drooling symptoms develop over shorter period of time (hours)), foreign body (acute onset, clear history), anaphylaxis (known allergy, urticaria, wheals), tracheitis (toxic child, croupy cough, no drooling), infectious mononucleosis (due to marked tonsillar swelling), diphtheria (rare but important, always check immunisation status).

E: Commonly affects children from 6 months to 5 years old. Occurs in the winter months and children may have repeated episodes.

H: **Coryza:** symptoms preceded by 1–3 days of coryza +/− fever.
Laryngitis: barking croupy cough and hoarse voice.
Tracheitis: onset of stridor (seal-like yelp) 1–2 days after cough.
Bronchitis: ↑respiratory effort as infection spreads down bronchial tree.

E: Examine the child in a calm environment with minimal disturbance.
Classification of severity of croup to determine management:

Mild croup	**Moderate croup**	**Severe croup**
No stridor Normal RR No recession Normal HR Normal O_2 sats Normal GCS	Stridor at rest, audible with stethoscope Mild recession Normal/↑RR AE decreased but easily audible ↑HR O_2 sat > 93% Normal GCS	Stridor at rest, audible without stethoscope Laboured breathing; tachypnoea + recession AE decreased and difficult to hear ↑HR O_2 sats < 93% Altered GCS Cyanosis

Do not examine the child's throat as it may precipitate acute airway obstruction.

P: **Macro:** mucosal inflammation and ↑secretions affecting the larynx, trachea, and bronchi. Narrowing of the subglottic area causes stridor and is potentially dangerous in young children because of their narrow trachea.

I: Blood tests are seldom taken as aim is to cause least distress to child and because croup is a clinical diagnosis.

M: **Mild croup:** most resolve spontaneously and may be managed conservatively at home. Humidity is popular with parents but is of unproven value. Paracetamol PRN mg be used for symptomatic relief and to ↓temperature.
Moderate croup: oral steroids (dexamethasone/prednisolone) or nebulised budesonide has been shown to shorten duration and severity of disease. Observe for 2–4 hs post administration of steroids to watch for deterioration.
Severe croup: nebulised adrenaline (5 ml of 1:1000) with O_2 may be used as a temporary measure as is effective in reducing upper airways oedema but watch for rebound obstruction. Treat with steroids as in moderate croup. May require intubation and admission to PICU.

C: Upper airway obstruction may be fatal.

P: Duration usually 2–3 days, occasionally 2–3 weeks. 2–5% of children hospitalised for croup require intubation.

D: Testis that has failed to descend from the abdomen into the scrotum after 1 year of age. **Types of cryptorchidism:**

(1) **True undescended testes:** the testes are found within the normal path of descent with a patent processus vaginalis; may be found intra-abdominally or within the inguinal canal.

(2) **Maldescended testes:** testes have descended through the inguinal canal but are positioned in the SC tissue outside the scrotum, e.g. perineum, femoral, suprapubic regions.

A: Precise cause has not been proven. 3 main areas of development have been researched: the hypothalamus–pituitary–gonadal axis, the epididymis, the gubernaculum and genitofemoral nerve.

A/R: Preterm infants, low birth weight, hydrocoele, hypospadias, inguinal hernia (always present with true undescended testes and common with ectopic testes), if bilateral may be due to hypopituitarism.

E: 0.8% of boys >1 year.

H: Usually asymptomatic, picked up during child health surveillance.

E: Examine relaxed child in a warm room. The most common location of the cryptorchid testes is in the inguinal canal (72%), followed by prescrotal (20%), and abdominal (8%) locations. Examine for inguinal hernias.

DD:

(1) Retractile testis: often bilateral, normal condition commonly seen in prepubertal boys.

(2) Congenital absence: rare; only in 4% of patients who clinically have an undescended testis.

(3) Atrophied testis: usually 2° to torsion.

P: See **A**.

I: **Diagnosis is usually clinical.**

USS pelvis: detects cryptorchid testis below the level of the internal inguinal ring; however, cannot detect intra-abdominal testes.

MRI/CT: can detect intra-abdominal testes.

Hormonal screen: performed in bilateral cryptorchidism.

(1) **Gonadotrophins:** ↑FSH/LH indicate a congenitally anorchid patient as there is a lack of negative feedback by testosterone. ↓/Normal FSH/LH levels may indicate functioning gonadal tissue.

(2) **HCG stimulation:** a rise in testosterone levels after HCG stimulation indicates functioning testicular tissue.

Chromosomal testing: performed in bilateral cryptorchidism.

M: **Medical: HCG;** may be used to induce testicular descent in bilateral cryptorchidism when the testes are near the scrotum, success rate 10%.

Surgical: orchidopexy age <2 years. Orchidectomy in intra-abdominal testes or severely atrophied testes. Testicular prostheses are available.

C: **Infertility:**

If uncorrected: unilateral cryptorchidism has a similar rate of infertility to the general population. In bilateral cryptorchidism almost all adults are infertile.

If corrected: in bilateral cryptorchidism 67% adults are infertile.

Malignancy: 20–44% ↑ risk of testicular tumour (seminoma in 60%) at age 30–40 years. Risk ↑ in uncorrected intra-abdominal testes and ↓ with surgical correction at <8 years.

Testicular torsion.

P: Good with appropriate surgical intervention.

Cystic fibrosis (CF)

D: Autosomal recessive condition characterised by recurrent lung infections, malabsorption, and failure to thrive.

A: **Common genotype (70–80%):** phenylalanine deletion at position 508 (ΔF508) gives rise to a defective gene on chromosome 7 q. There are up to 900 known mutations of this gene. Defective gene codes for abnormal transport protein (CFTR) in the cell membrane.

A/R: Obstructive azoospermia (may occur in some CF individuals without other symptoms).

E: 1/2500 Caucasian live births. 1/25 carrier rate in Caucasians.

H: **Neonatal:** meconium ileus (bowel obstruction by thick meconium).
Infancy: recurrent chest infections, steatorrhoea, failure to thrive, developmental delay.
Older children: asthma, allergic bronchopulmonary aspergillosis (episodic wheeze, low-grade fever, brown sputum), recurrent sinusitis.

E: **Signs of malnutrition:** ↓muscle mass progressing to gross wasting, protuberant abdomen.
Respiratory: hyperinflation (air trapping), coarse crepitations, expiratory rhonchi.
Others: jaundice, early digital clubbing, nasal polyps.

I: **Sweat test:** gold standard; sweat Cl^- of > 50 mmol/L and Na^{2+} of >60 mmol/L by pilocarpine iontophoresis, weight of sweat >100 mg on 2 occasions. Newer methods (macroduct) require less.
Lung function: obstructive picture with air trapping and hyperinflation (↓FEV1, ↑TLC).
Guthrie's test: ↑serum immunoreactive trypsin (neonatal screening is being introduced in the UK).
Antenatal tests: 1st trimester CVS (95% sensitivity).
2nd trimester ↓intestinal ALP in amniotic fluid (90% sensitivity).

P: **Genetic:** defective CFTR acts as cAMP chloride channel blocker. ↓Cl^- transport accompanied by ↓Na^+ and H_2O transport across epithelial cells results in dehydrated viscous secretions causing luminal obstruction, destruction, and scarring of exocrine glands.
Respiratory: lung is normal at birth but as it matures, mucous gland hyperplasia and thick viscid mucous is formed in the small airways. Patients are predisposed to chronic infection with *Staphylococcus aureus*, *Haemophilus influenzae*, and *Pseudomonas* which leads to areas of fibrosis, consolidation, and bronchiectasis.
Pancreatic: exocrine enzyme insufficiency causes malabsorption and steatorrhoea.

M: **Multidisciplinary approach:**
Respiratory:
(1) Most children are on prophylaxis for *Staphylococcus aureus.*
(2) 80% of CF patients are chronically infected by adolescence with *pseudomonas*. This is treated with nebulised antibiotics (colomycin +/− gentamicin/tobramycin) and intermittent courses of IV antibiotics to decrease size of colony (usually every 3 months).
(3) Allergic bronchopulmonary aspergillosis; treated with steroids +/− itraconazole.
(4) ↑Airway responsiveness presents with asthma-like symptoms. Treated with bronchodilators +/− inhaled steroids if responsive.
(5) Nebulised recombinant human DNAase acts as a mucolytic.

Nutritional: ↑calorie, ↑protein diet for ↑energy requirements and malabsorption often with overnight supplementation. Some CF patients have a gastrostomy inserted to facilitate ↑calorie intake. Enteric-coated pancreatic enzyme (e.g. Creon) and fat-soluble vitamin supplementation.

Immunisations: usual schedule + pneumococcal, influenza.
Physiotherapy: $>2\times$ daily, depending on sputum produced. Swimming is an ideal sport. Should be maintained even when well.
Heart-lung transplant: if lung function deteriorates to $<30\%$ predicted best.
Gene therapy: viral vectors/liposomes to deliver normal copies of the CF gene to make the CFTR protein. Still at research stage.

C: **Respiratory:** pneumonia, cor pulmonale, pneumothorax, haemoptysis.
GI: cirrhosis, portal hypertension, distal intestinal obstruction syndrome – viscid mucofaeculent material obstructs the bowel.
Endocrine: DM, ↓fertility, 99% of males are infertile due to obstruction and abnormal development of vas deferens. Females are often subfertile but there have been many successful pregnancies.
Psychological/behavioural problems: due to compromised lifestyle and fear of death.

P: Most sufferers now survive into adult life (median survival 40 years). Patients with pancreatic insufficiency or colonisation with pseudomonas have a poorer prognosis.

Delayed puberty

D: Failure to exhibit the physical signs of puberty within the expected time period in the normal population.

Males: absence of testicular enlargement by 14 years.

Females: absence of thelarche (breast development) by 13 years and/or menarche by 16 years.

A: **Normal gonadotrophins (LH, FSH):**

(1) Constitutional delay: due to late activation of the hypothalamic–pituitary–gonadal axis, delay is synchronous for height and bone age.
(2) Chronic illness: inflammatory bowel disease, CF, renal disease, severe asthma.
(3) AN, starvation, excess physical training (ballet, athletes).
(4) Deprivation (emotional abuse, neglect).

Hypergonadotropic hypogonadism/unresponsive gonad:

(1) Congenital: Turner syndrome (45X karyotype), Klinefelter syndrome (47XXY).
(2) Steroid hormone enzyme deficiency.
(3) Acquired gonadal damage: chemotherapy, radiotherapy, trauma, torsion, autoimmune.

Hypogonadotropic hypogonadism/failure of hypothalamic or pituitary function:

(1) Hypothalamo–pituitary disease: panhypopituitarism, intracranial tumours (craniopharyngioma).
(2) Kallmann syndrome (LHRH deficiency, anosmia).
(3) Hypothyroidism (acquired).
(4) Idiopathic.

A/R: Family history in constitutional delay.

E: **Turner syndrome:** 1/2500 live births.

Klinefelter syndrome: 1–2/1000 live births.

Idiopathic hypogonadotropic hypogonadism: 1/50 000 females, 1/10 000 males.

Physiological or constitutional delay: 1/200. M > F.

H: Elicit family history, symptoms of chronic disease (failure to thrive, lethargy), and social history.

E: **General:** full examination to detect any indication of underlying disease, neurological signs (fundi, visual fields), dysmorphic features.

Testicular size: orchidometer; 4 ml at 10–14 years, 12 ml at 12–17 years.

Tanner stages of puberty:

Male genital stages

(1) Preadolescent.
(2) Lengthening of penis.
(3) ↑Length and circumference.
(4) Glans penis, scrotal darkening.
(5) Adult genitalia.

Female breast stages

(1) Prepubertal.
(2) Breast bud.
(3) Juvenile smooth contour.
(4) Areola/nipple projects above breast.
(5) Same shape nipple and breast.

Pubic hair changes in males and females

(1) Preadolescent, no sexual hair.
(2) Long downy hair along labia/base of penis.
(3) Dark, coarser, curlier hair.
(4) Filling out towards adult distribution.
(5) Adult in quantity and type, with spread to medial thigh.

P: See **A**.

I: **Bloods:** TFTs, LH/FSH/androgen/oestrogen levels.
Karyotype: chromosomal abnormalities.
Radiology: determination of bone age (delayed in constitutional delay), USS pelvis to assess uterine size and endometrial thickness, cranial MRI if signs/symptoms suspicious of intracranial tumour.

M: **Paediatric endocrinologist referral:** management involves primarily education, reassurance, patience (especially constitutional delay) and treatment of any underlying cause. Induction of hormone treatment should be at the patient's and family's choice.
Females: oestrogen replacement therapy is the treatment of choice. This can be administered orally or transdermally. After 12–18 months of unopposed oestrogen therapy or after vaginal bleeding occurs progesterone should be added.
Males: hormonal replacement with testosterone IM (monthly) or PO (daily).

C: Individual conditions but also psychosocial, including poor self-esteem, reduced academic performance and socialising with peers.

P: Dependent on underlying pathology.

Depression

D: **Major depressive disorder:** defined in children and adolescents as in adults; low mood, anhedonia (inability to enjoy), and feeling of worthlessness for two or more weeks.
Adjustment disorder: less severe depression due to life event (parental separation/loss).

A: **Genetic:** depressed children are more likely to have a parent with an affective disorder.
Environmental: poor support network, lack of friends, isolation.
Systemic disease: anaemia, postviral syndrome (e.g. EBV), hypothyroidism, chronic illness.

A/R: **Associated:** family history, substance abuse, neglect, family break-up, personal loss, learning disability.
Related: anxiety disorder, behavioural disorder, dysthymic disorder, and cyclothymia.

E: Prevalence rises with age; up to 2.5% of children and 8% of adolescents. M : F equal during childhood, but females are more likely to suffer depression during and after adolescence.

H&E: Manifestation of depression in children is affected by their developmental stage and ability to identify and communicate internal emotions.
Children and adolescents will often use other means of expression such as:
(1) Somatisation with frequent vague, nonspecific physical complaints.
(2) Poor academic performance, truantism.
(3) Being bored, lack of interest in anything.
(4) Disorganised or reckless behaviour.
(5) Separation anxiety, loss of interest in friends, social withdrawal.
(6) Outbursts of shouting, complaining, unexplained irritability, or crying.
(7) Alcohol or substance abuse.
(8) Hitting, biting, scratching, self-harm, suicide.
Children and adolescents are less likely to present with biological symptoms such as reduced appetite, insomnia and early morning waking, or psychotic disturbances.
In children depression is often interspersed with periods of relative normality.

P: Reduction in serotonergic and NA nerve transmission within the brain is thought to contribute to depression. There is a reduction in activity within the prefrontal cortex, which may have a part in 5-HT and NA neuron regulation.

I: **Bloods:** FBC, LFTs, TFTs, U&E if clinical suspicion of systemic disease.

M: **Medical:** SSRIs (e.g. fluoxetine) have been shown to be effective in treating children and adolescents.
CBT: effective in adolescent depression.

C: **Self-harm:** a desperate attempt to draw attention to a perceived irresolvable situation. High rate of recurrence (note – majority are *not* clinically depressed).
Suicide: most common in adolescent boys, ↑risk if combined with alcohol/substance abuse.

P: Untreated symptoms often extend 7–9 months. Up to 40% of children who have a major depressive episode are likely to have a relapse within 2 years.

Developmental dysplasia of the hip (DDH)

D: Failure of development of the normal hip joint after delivery.

A: Due to ligamentous laxity from ↑circulating maternal oestrogen.

A/R: Family history (1st degree relative in 20%), firstborn (smaller uterus), oligohydramnios (foetal compression syndrome), breech delivery, Caesarean section, neuromuscular disorders.

E: Most common musculoskeletal abnormality in neonates after accessory digits; 1–2/1000 live births. M : F = 1 : 6.
Commoner in Caucasians.

H: Elicit family history and any risk factors.

E: With a relaxed child the hip and knee are flexed to 90°, the thumbs of the examiner are placed on the medial proximal thigh, and the long fingers are placed over the greater trochanter.
Barlow's manoeuvre: the hip is adducted while pushing the thigh posteriorly. In a positive Barlow test, the hip is felt to go out of the socket and is therefore 'dislocatable'. The dislocation is confirmed by performing Ortolani's manoeuvre to relocate the hip.
Note: Hip manoeuvres should not be performed frequently as they can cause DDH themselves.
Ortolani's manoeuvre: the contralateral hip is held still while the thigh of the hip being tested is abducted and gently pulled anteriorly. In a positive Ortolani test, the femoral head can be pushed back with the fingers over the posterior rim of the acetabulum into the cavity. An audible clunk can sometimes be heard when this occurs.
Other physical signs:
(1) Diminished movement on the affected side.
(2) Asymmetry in leg positions.
(3) Asymmetry of the thigh fat folds.
(4) At > 3/12 asymmetry of rotation of the leg and apparent shortening of the affected leg.

P: Hips are not dislocated *in utero*; hence the hip is relatively normal. Following dislocation acetabular dysplasia and maldirection, excessive femoral anteversion (torsion), and contractures of the hip muscle develop.

I: **USS hip:** shows relationship of the femoral head to the acetabulum and the existence of any acetabular dysplasia; has a high false positive rate in infants < 6 weeks.
X-ray hip: useful if > 4 months as there is sufficient ossification of the upper femur and acetabulum.

M: **Supportive:** Pavlik harness adduction splints until 5–6 months.
Surgical correction: surgical release of the hip adductor and iliopsoas may be required if diagnosis occurs late (> 6 months). Closed reduction is the preferred method. After 18 months open reduction with femoral and/or pelvic osteotomy may be required to correct severe deformities.

C: **Iatrogenic:** skin irritation from reduction devices, 1–5% incidence of avascular necrosis of the femoral head with Pavlik harness splinting.
Long-term: osteoarthritis of the hip.

P: Almost always treated successfully with external splints. Older ages of diagnosis are associated with worse outcome. If untreated can be severely disabling.

Diabetes mellitus (Type I) (DM)

D: DM is a metabolic disorder characterised by hyperglycaemia as a result of the absence of insulin secretion (Type I) or insulin resistance (Type II). Most children are Type I; hence this page concentrates on Type I. There is, however, an ↑ of Type II DM in children especially in westernised countries due to rising incidence in obesity in children (see chapter).

A: **Genetic:** 50% concordance in monozygotic twins. 3% risk with maternal and 6% risk with paternal DM.
Environmental: viral infections; probably by initiating or modifying an autoimmune process.

A/R: Human leucocyte antigen DR-3 and DR-4, autoimmune disorders such as hypothyroidism.

E: **Incidence is rising:** 11.7–18.7/10 000/year (1978–97) in urban Yorkshire (age 0–14).
Peak age of onset: 4–6 years and 10–14 years (commonest).
There is considerable racial and geographical variation. M : F = 1.08 : 1.

H&E: **General:** polyuria (nocturnal enuresis/persistently wet nappies/nappy rash), polydipsia, weight loss, recurrent infections, necrobiosis lipoidica (well-demarcated, red atrophic area usually on lower leg).
DKA: abdominal pain, vomiting, dehydration, drowsiness progressing to coma, Kussmaul's respiration (rapid deep breathing) 2° to acidosis, acetone breath.
Hypoglycaemia (usually due to insulin treatment): sweating, tremor, palpitations, irritability, *late* – seizures, coma.

P: Autoimmune destruction of β cells of pancreas, with the presence of islet cell antibodies and glutamic acid decarboxylase antibodies. Insulin deficiency → ↓cellular uptake of glucose, ↑gluconeogenesis (from protein breakdown), and ketone production (from fatty acid breakdown).

I: **Urinalysis:** ketonuria, glycosuria.
Blood glucose: random > 11.0 mmol/L; fasting > 7.0 mmol/L.
Glycosylated Hb: $HbA_{1c} > 7.5\%$.
DKA: low blood bicarbonate, ↓pH, heavy ketonuria.
Hypoglycaemia: plasma glucose < 2.5 mmol/L.

M: **Parental and patient education:** about nature of DM, recognition of hypoglycaemia, insulin regime and technique, ↑insulin requirements in illness (sick day rules) and maintenance of active lifestyle.
Total insulin requirement: DNA recombinant human insulin 0.5–1 unit/kg/day in prepubertal children. Insulin resistance in adolescents may require 2 units/kg/day.
Insulin regimes: If b.d., short-acting (soluble, regular) insulin combined with intermediate-acting insulin before breakfast (two-thirds daily dose) and before dinner (one-third daily dose); usually given in combined solution by PEN. Many children now start t.d.s. regime; q.d.s. regime may be used in older children using short-acting insulin before main meals and an intermediate insulin before bedtime to provide more flexibility.
Insulin pump therapy: ↑numbers of children are using continuous SC insulin infusion using long-acting insulin glargine and bolus doses at meal times.
Blood glucose monitoring: aim for 4–6 mmol/L.
Diet: high fibre, ↓refined carbohydrate but ↑complex carbohydrate consumption.
Psychological impact of chronic disease: due to restrictive lifestyle and diet.

Medic Alert bracelet/necklace.

DKA:

Appropriate fluid resuscitation with IV normal saline.

↓

Insulin sliding scale: short-acting soluble insulin via syringe driver (0.25 units/kg/h).

↓

Hourly U&E + K^+ replacement on passing urine (plasma K^+ falls as K^+ enters cells with treatment).

↓

Switch to IV dextrose saline when glucose levels fall to <12 mmol/L.

Hypoglycaemia:

Mild: food, e.g. apple/sandwich.

Moderate: oral glucose-rich drink + subsequent complex carbohydrate.

Severe: intrabuccal hypostop (complex glucose gel); rarely IV dextrose or IM glucagon is required.

C: **Acute:** hypoglycaemia, hyperglycaemia, and DKA.

Chronic: microvascular (retinopathy, neuropathy, nephropathy, cataracts) and macrovascular (IHD, stroke) disease.

P: DKA in young children and adolescents may be missed which may → fatalities, usually from subsequent cerebral oedema during treatment for DKA. DM is associated with morbidity and mortality from complications that can be reduced by good glycaemic control.

Down syndrome (trisomy 21)

D: Condition resulting from the presence of 3 chromosome 21s instead of 2.

A: **Nondisjunction at meiosis (95%):** extra maternal chromosome, i.e. karyotype 47XX+21 or 47XY+21. Incidence of trisomy 21 due to nondisjunction rises with ↑maternal age especially >35 years and is independent of paternal age.

Robertsonian translocation (4%): chromosome 21 usually translocated onto chromosome 14.

Mosaicism (1%): some cells normal, some trisomy 21 due to nondisjunction during mitosis after fertilisation; usually less severely affected.

A/R: **CHD (40%):** AVSD, VSD, ASD, Fallot's tetralogy, PDA.

GI: anal, oesophageal, and duodenal atresia (one-third of infants with duodenal atresia have Down syndrome), Hirschsprung disease.

Chronic secretory otitis media: gives rise to conductive hearing loss.

Others: recurrent respiratory infections, cataracts, squints, hypothyroidism.

E: 1/700 live births. Most common genetic cause of learning difficulties.

Risk increases with maternal age: < 30 ys (1/2000), 30 ys (1/1300), 35 ys (1/400), 40 ys (1/90).

Risk of recurrence: 1/200 if >35 and 2× age-specific rate if <35.

H: Most cases of Down syndrome are now diagnosed antenatally (see **I**).

E: **General:** neonatal hypotonia, short stature.

Developmental: mild to moderate learning disability (IQ 25–70, with social skills exceeding other intellectual functions).

Craniofacial: microcephaly, brachycephaly (shortness of skull), round face, epicanthic folds, upward sloping palpebral fissures, protruding tongue, flat nasal bridge, small ears, excess skin at back of neck, atlantoaxial instability.

Eyes: strabismus, nystagmus, Brushfield's spots in iris, cataracts.

Limbs: 5th finger clinodactyly, single palmar crease, wide gap between 1st and 2nd toes, hyperflexible joints in infants.

Cardiovascular: murmurs dependent on CHD, arrhythmias, CHF.

GI: vomiting (atresias), constipation (Hirschsprung disease).

P: See **A**.

I: **Antenatal screening:** maternal age is combined with the 'triple test' at 19 weeks on maternal serum: AFP (↓), unconjugated oestriol (↓), HCG (↑), and nuchal USS, to predict risk of having trisomy 21.

Confirmation of diagnosis: antenatal examination of foetal cells from amniocentesis or CVS, postnatal chromosomal analysis.

Screening for complications: echo, TFTs, hearing and vision assessment and follow-up.

M: **Multidisciplinary approach:** parental education and support, genetic counselling, IQ testing, and appropriate educational input.

Medical: antibiotics in recurrent respiratory infections, thyroid hormone in hypothyroidism.

Surgical: congenital heart defects, oesophageal/duodenal atresia.

C: ↓Fertility. 15× normal risk of leukaemia. Most develop Alzheimer's disease by 40 years of age as gene coding for amyloid protein found in Alzheimer's disease is located on chromosome 21.

P: **Antenatal:** 75% of trisomy 21 spontaneously abort.

Childhood: 15–20% of children with Down syndrome die <5 years usually due to severe CHD.

Adulthood: 50% now survive > 50 years but undergo premature ageing.

Duchenne/Becker muscular dystrophy

D: X-linked recessive degenerative muscle disorders, characterised by progressive muscle weakness and wasting of variable distribution and severity.
DMD: rapidly progressive form of muscular dystrophy.
BMD: slowly progressive form of muscular dystrophy.

A: **DMD:** caused by gene mutations on Xp21 which result in the absence of dystrophin (< 5% of normal). Two-thirds are inherited, one-third are de novo mutations. Dystrophin is a protein that forms part of a membrane-spanning protein complex of the muscle sarcolemma. This connects the cytoskeleton to the basal lamina.
BMD: exon deletions exist in the dystrophin gene Xp21 in 70% of cases. Dystrophin levels are 30–80% of normal. It is thought that abnormal translation of the dystrophin gene produces abnormal but partially functional dystrophin.

A/R: Family history.

E: **DMD:** the most common type of muscular dystrophy; 1/3000 live male births
BMD: 3–6/100 000 live male births.

H: **DMD:** the child appears healthy at birth. Onset of symptoms is from age 1–6 with a waddling gait, toe-walking, difficulty running, climbing stairs, or getting up from a seated or lying position. By age 10 braces are required for walking, by age 12 most children are wheelchair-bound. In 20% there is associated learning disability.
BMD: symptoms appear around age 10 and are a milder version of those in DMD.

E: **Distribution of muscle weakness:** symmetrical; more prominent in the pelvic and shoulder girdle.
Calf muscle pseudohypertrophy: results from excessive adipose replacement of muscle fibres.
Gowers' sign: child uses hands against thighs, pushing down on them, in order to overcome proximal muscle and pelvic girdle weakness to stand up from seated position on floor.

P: Variation in muscle fibre size, segmental necrosis of fibre groups. Initially, fibre regeneration occurs, but this fails and → loss of muscle and replacement by adipose cells and connective tissue.

I: **Bloods:** high levels of creatinine kinase are present in the serum from birth.
EMG: establishes the myopathic nature and excludes neurogenic causes of muscle weakness.
Muscle biopsy and immunostaining for dystrophin.
Genetic testing: identification of the specific mutation or defect is carried out in specialised centres.

M: **Multidisciplinary approach:**
Medical:
(1) Oral steroids have been shown to have a beneficial effect in controlled studies, helping to maintain mobility for a further 2–3 years.
(2) Early detection of a cardiomyopathy enables early appropriate management.
(3) Respiratory care and assisted respiration in the form of non-invasive intermittent PPV may be required at a later stage.

Surgical: correction of contractures to maintain mobility and scoliosis to preserve lung function.
Orthopaedic/physiotherapy: moderate physical exercise, mobility aids, night splints, spinal supports.
Education: may require attendance to schools for children with physical disabilities and/or learning disability.

Genetic counselling of female family members: prenatal tests are 95% accurate using CVS for DNA typing.
Psychological: support and counselling for parent and child.

C: Loss of mobility, limb contractures, scoliosis, respiratory insufficiency and infection, dilated cardiomyopathy at >15 years. Side-effects of long-term steroids.

P: Progressive muscle weakness and heart failure.
DMD: respiratory and cardiac failure is the main cause of death. Few live beyond their late twenties.
BMD: disease develops later and less rapidly. Most patients walk beyond 16 years of age and may maintain this into adulthood.

Encephalitis

D: Inflammation of the brain parenchyma.

A: **Viruses:** enteroviruses, HSV1, HSV2, VZV, arboviruses, adenoviruses, HIV, mumps (rare now due to immunisation), rubella, and rabies.
Post-measles: SSPE.

A/R: Foreign travel, measles, immunosuppression, active maternal HSV2 infection.

E: 1/100 000. **Peak age:** 3–8 months. Commonest in <4 years.

H: **General:** lethargy, poor feeding, irritability, hypotonia, behavioural change, vomiting.
Neurological: headache, drowsiness, confusion, photophobia, neck pain, seizures (focal fits suggestive of HSV encephalitis).
Associated: pharyngitis, conjunctivitis, and myositis.

E: **General:** fever, $\downarrow$GCS, positive Kernig's sign; pain on extension of the knee with hips and knees flexed whilst in a supine position.
Neurological: cranial nerve and motor abnormalities, ataxia (varicella-associated encephalitis).

P: **Infectious:** viruses enter into the blood stream during systemic febrile illness and affect several organs. There is further viral replication and subsequent invasion into the brain parenchyma with cell destruction, localised inflammation, swelling, and inflammation of the meninges. HSV probably reaches the brain directly via neuronal axons.
Post-infectious: immune-mediated reaction to viral antigens that $\rightarrow$ perivascular inflammation and demyelination.

I: **Bloods:** FBC, blood cultures, serum glucose, U&Es, serum and urine osmolalities.
LP for CSF: WCC; normal/$\uparrow$lymphocytes, protein; mildly $\uparrow$/normal, glucose: $\downarrow$/normal.
CSF microscopy: Gram stain, culture and sensitivity.
CSF PCR: HSV.
CSF serology: HSV antibody can be detected in the CSF in later stages.
Radiology: CT/MRI brain may show oedema, or focal lesions (particularly in the temporal lobes) with HSV encephalitis.
EEG: shows diffuse slow wave activity usually without focal changes.
ICP monitoring: may be required in severe cases.

M: **Empirical antibiotic therapy:** 3rd generation cephalosporin is indicated until bacterial meningitis is excluded.
Supportive: fluid resuscitation and correction of electrolyte imbalance, anticonvulsants for seizures, analgesia for headache.
Antivirals: all children with suspected encephalitis should initially be treated with acyclovir to cover the possibility of HSV encephalitis. Confirmed HSV encephalitis requires a 3-week course of IV acyclovir.
Follow-up: regular neurological and audiological assessment.
Prevention: MMR vaccine.

C: HSV encephalitis may cause hemiparesis, deafness, epilepsy, visual impairment, bilateral motor impairment, learning and language difficulties. Neurological deficits also occur following arbovirus and 2° viral infection in HIV patients.

P: Many cases of encephalitis make a full recovery; however, this is dependent on age, aetiology, and severity. There is a 70% mortality rate with untreated HSV encephalitis, and survivors often have severe neurological defects.

Epiglottitis, acute

D: An uncommon life-threatening emergency due to inflammation of the epiglottis causing upper respiratory airway obstruction.

A: Caused by infection with the bacterium Hib.

A/R: ↑Risk in the non-immunised child. However, immunisation does not provide complete protection.
DD of acute stridor: acute laryngotracheobronchitis (croup); child is less toxic, and develops over greater period of time (days), foreign body (acute onset, clear history), anaphylaxis (known allergy, wheals), infectious mononucleosis (due to marked tonsillar swelling), tracheitis (toxic child, croupy cough, no drooling), diphtheria (rare but important).

E: A rarer condition in the UK since introduction of the Hib vaccine. Affects mainly children aged 2–4 years.

H: **Sudden onset (3–6 hours):** very unwell child, fever, drooling due to inability to swallow because of pain in pharynx. Not usually hoarse, and rarely has a cough (to differentiate from croup/tracheitis).

E: **General:** ill, toxic-looking, pyrexial ($>38.5^\circ$C), tachycardia.
Specific signs:
(1) Difficulty breathing and stridor (harsh inspiratory noise).
(2) Unable to talk and swallow due to intensely painful throat.
(3) Drooling with characteristic sitting posture (sitting upright with the throat thrust forward).
Do not examine the child's throat or distress the child as this may precipitate acute airways obstruction.

P: **Macro:** typically the epiglottis looks cherry red and swollen due to inflammation from 2° acute bacterial infection.

I: **Take bloods only after intubation to prevent acute airways obstruction.**
Blood cultures: to determine bacteria.
ABG: to determine severity of respiratory compromise.

M: Keep child comfortable at all times; do not take away from mother, do not force to lie down.
Resuscitation:
Airway: give O_2; call for senior anaesthetist to intubate by gaseous induction.
Breathing: ensure good air entry to chest.
Circulation: IV access, bloods, colloid if shocked (20 ml/kg).
Antibiotics: 3rd generation cephalosporin IV as Hib strains are resistant to ampicillin and chloramphenicol, continue for 5 days.
Prophylaxis: with rifampicin is offered to close household contacts.
Once stabilised transfer to PICU.

C: Acute airway obstruction.

P: With prompt diagnosis and management most children recover within 3–5 days. Expect to extubate after 24–48 h. There is significant risk of death or brain injury if obstruction occurs.

D: Two or more unprovoked seizures. A seizure is defined as an abnormal, disorderly discharging of the brain's nerve cells, resulting in a temporary disturbance of motor, sensory, or mental function.

A: **1°:** idiopathic in most cases; many have positive family history.

2°: head trauma, encephalitis, meningitis, CNS tumours, hypoxic–ischaemic injury, intrauterine infections, cerebral dysgenesis (e.g. cerebral palsy), and specific aetiologies (e.g. TS).

A/R: See **A**.

E: 1% of children suffer from epilepsy.

H: **Generalised seizures:** large part of cortex is involved, consciousness is impaired:

- **Absence seizures (petit mal):** onset usually between 4 and 12 years. Short episodes (< 20 s) during which the child stares or blinks, with no apparent awareness of the surroundings. Can occur >100×/day. There is no aura or post-ictal phase. May present as 'daydreaming' in class, or ↓ in school performance.
- **Myoclonic seizures:** sudden brief muscle contractions; often cluster within a few minutes. If they evolve into rhythmic jerking movements, they are classified as evolving into a clonic seizure.
- **Clonic seizures:** rhythmic, jerking movements that simultaneously involve the upper and lower extremities.
- **Tonic seizures:** sudden onset tonic extension or flexion of the head, trunk, and/or extremities for several seconds.
- **GTCS (grand mal):** generalised tonic extension lasting for a few seconds followed by clonic rhythmic movements and a prolonged post-ictal phase (confusion/somnolence). Often associated with urinary or faecal incontinence.
- **Atonic seizures:** consist of brief loss of postural tone, often resulting in falls and injuries. This seizure type occurs in people with significant neurologic abnormalities.

Partial seizures: involve only a part of the brain and therefore only a part of the body/mind:

- **Simple partial seizures:** occurrence of a seizure with preservation of consciousness. Many kinds of simple partial seizures exist, including sensory, motor, autonomic, and psychic experiences. Motor (asynchronous tonic or clonic movements) dysfunction, is initially localised to one area of the body but may move to different parts of the body as the seizure is propagated.
- **Complex partial seizures:** similar to simple partial seizure; however, consciousness is impaired and episode is followed by post-ictal phase.
- **Partial seizures with 2° generalisation:** focal seizure is followed by GTCS.

Epilepsy syndromes:

- **Infantile spasms:** affect infants aged 4–8 months. Clusters of myoclonic spasms; classical 'Salaam' attack where child jerks forward with arms flexed and hands extended. Often associated with learning disability.
- **Lennox–Gastaut syndrome:** affects children aged 1–3 years. Characterised by multiple seizure types (tonic-axial, atonic, and absence seizures), developmental regression, and learning disability.
- **Benign partial rolandic epilepsy:** affects children aged 4–10 years. Clonic seizures affecting face and upper limbs usually during sleep; may progress to GTCS.

- **Juvenile myoclonic epilepsy:** affects adolescents; idiopathic generalised epileptic syndrome characterised by myoclonic jerks, GTCS, and sometimes absence seizures, usually on awakening.

Status epilepticus: a seizure (usually GTCS) lasting longer than 30 min or repeated seizures without a return to normal in between. Requires urgent intervention to terminate seizure (see Appendix).

E: General and neurological examination to rule out specific aetiologies (TS) and focal neurological signs.

P: Imbalance between excitatory and inhibitory neurotransmission resulting in high-frequency burst activity seen as spike and wave on EEG. Seizure propagates if sufficient surrounding neurons are recruited.

I: **EEG:** epileptiform spike and wave activity correlates with different forms of epilepsy. (e.g. hypsarrhythmia in infantile spasms).
MRI: to rule out underlying pathology, e.g. glial tumour.
Lumbar puncture: if infective cause suspected.

M: **Long-term management of epilepsy in order of preference:**
Generalised epilepsy:

- Absence seizures: sodium valproate, lamotrigine, or ethosuximide, exacerbated by carbamazepine.
- Myoclonic: sodium valproate, lamotrigine, clobazam, or clonazepam.
- Tonic-clonic: sodium valproate, carbamazepine, or lamotrigine.

Partial epilepsy: carbamazepine, sodium valproate, gabapentin, topiramate, lamotrigine, or vigabatrin.
Epilepsy syndromes:

- Infantile spasms: ACTH, prednisolone, vigabatrin.
- Lennox–Gastaut syndrome: lamotrigine, topiramate, vigabatrin. Corpus callosotomy in refractory cases.
- Benign partial rolandic epilepsy: carbamazepine for problematic or daytime seizures only.
- Juvenile myoclonic epilepsy: sodium valproate.

Education: explain nature of epilepsy to parent and child.
Advice: aim is to give child utmost confidence and independence possible. Avoid precipitating factors such as alcohol, sleep deprivation, drugs. Supervision when in swimming pools or baths.

C: Impaired neurological development, poor school performance, learning disability.

P: Patients with epilepsy have a mortality rate 2–3× that of the general population. (SUDEP)
GTCS: usually require lifelong treatment with anticonvulsants.
Absence seizures: usually undergo spontaneous remission during adolescence.
Infantile spasms: poor outcome usually → chronic epilepsy and impaired neurological development.
Lennox–Gastaut syndrome: often resistant to therapy and is associated with continued seizures during adult life.
Benign partial rolandic epilepsy: usually undergo spontaneous remission during adolescence.
Juvenile myoclonic epilepsy: require lifelong treatment, not associated with intellectual impairment.

D: Exomphalos and gastroschisis are both congenital anterior wall defects.

A: **Exomphalos:** failure of the midgut to return to the abdomen. A defect at the umbilicus causes the abdominal contents to protrude through the umbilical ring. This protrusion is covered with a transparent sac that is composed of amniotic membrane and peritoneum. In large defects the liver will also protrude.

Gastroschisis: literally means split stomach. There is a defect in the anterior abdominal wall adjacent to the umbilicus, usually to the right. At the site of this defect there is a protrusion of loops of bowel matted together, with no covering.

A/R: The presence of other abnormalities is common with exomphalos, especially Beckwith–Wiedemann syndrome (exomphalos, macroglossia, and gigantism) and trisomy 13 and 18. There are usually none associated with gastroschisis.

E: **Exomphalos:** 1/3000 live births.
Gastroschisis: 1/5000 live births.

H: The defect is usually detected antenatally through USS. The baby can therefore be delivered at a paediatric surgical unit and the parents forewarned about the need for surgery.

E: A protrusion is seen in the neonate, either in the umbilical region or to the right of it.

Exomphalos: widening of the umbilical cord with the protrusion. Care needs to be taken to avoid clamping across the lesion when the umbilical cord is clamped.

Gastroschisis: matted collection of loops of bowel, which are red in appearance, protruding from the anterior abdominal wall.

P: Congenital abnormality giving rise to defect in the anterior abdominal wall.

I: **USS:** both of these defects are usually detected antenatally.

M: **General supportive measures:** NG tube is passed and aspirated frequently, IV access is established and dextrose infusion started.

Dehydration/protein loss: the abdomen of affected infants should be wrapped in cling film to minimise fluid and heat loss. Colloid support is often needed to replace protein loss.

Surgery: the majority of lesions can be repaired by 1° closure of the abdomen. With larger lesions a Silastic sac is sewn over and used to return the abdominal contents to the peritoneal cavity within 1–2 weeks.

C: Dehydration and protein loss (↑risk in gastroschisis).

P: Good with antenatal diagnosis and adequate supportive and surgical management in a specialised centre. In exomphalos the prognosis can be made worse by the presence of other coexisting abnormalities.

Faecal soiling (encopresis)

D: Voluntary or involuntary passage of faeces after the age at which faecal continence is considered normal (> 4 years).

A: **1°encopresis:** when bowel control has never been established. Occurs in a disorganised family, understaffed institution, or in children with learning difficulties.

2° encopresis: when bowel control has been established for at least 6 months before soiling occurs. This is usually caused by emotional, physical, or iatrogenic factors.

Emotional causes:

- **Regressive encopresis:** the child returns to an earlier stage of development 2° to an upsetting life event.
- **Aggressive encopresis:** occurs in the presence of a bad relationship between a child and parent/sibling/carer (act of rebellion).

Physical causes: anal fissures and rashes that cause pain on defaecation. Constipation may also lead to pain on defaecation with retention of faeces, distention of the rectum and subsequent overflow diarrhoea.

Iatrogenic causes: dietary manipulation and overly aggressive management of constipation with laxatives and enemas.

A/R: Child's emotional state, and factors affecting this, e.g. sexual abuse, behavioural problems, and enuresis.

E: 3/100 children aged 5 years, 2/100 children aged 7–8 years, 1/100 boys aged 12 years; M : F = 4 : 1.

H: **Detailed history from the family and child:** is it 1° or 2° encopresis? What toileting skills have been achieved? When is the child most likely to soil? What are the motions like? Could there be any physical cause? Are there any emotional influences? Does the parent/carer praise progress made or offer the child encouragement?

E: May have abdominal distension. Inspection of the anus and digital rectal examination should be performed to exclude fissures or tears. Observe family interactions.

P: See **A**.

I: Usually none are required.

M: **Physical causes:** should be excluded on examination and treated if present.

If no physical cause is found, encopresis is a positive diagnosis and should be treated as such.

Regular toileting: can be initiated by using laxative (e.g. senna) at night to encourage a motion in the morning after breakfast (gastrocolic reflex). This may require reorganisation of the family schedule so that the family are up in time to have breakfast, and the child then has 10 min alone on the toilet (with no one asking whether the child managed to pass a motion).

Parental education: techniques to reinforce good behaviour, with encouragement during periods of relapse.

Child education: exploration of the child's self-perception and its relationship with soiling; behavioural programmes can help the child to recognise own body signals.

C: If untreated can → low self-esteem with associated social consequences.

P: Depends on the underlying cause. It is unusual for encopresis to persist beyond middle teenage years.

Failure to thrive

D: Failure to thrive is a description applied to children whose current weight or rate of weight gain is significantly below that of other children of similar age and sex.
One-off assessment: weight below the 2nd centile.
Continual assessment: crossing 2 centile channels for weight.

A: **Functional (most common cause):**
(1) **Nutritional neglect:** poor understanding of feeding techniques, exclusion diets.
(2) **Emotional neglect:** stimulus deprivation.
(3) **Abuse:** physical, sexual, Munchausen syndrome by proxy.
(4) **Psychiatric:** AN, depression.

Organic:
(1) **Feeding difficulties:** mechanical (cleft palate disorders), neurological (CP).
(2) **Poor retention of food:** GORD, cow's milk protein intolerance.
(3) **Poor absorption of food:** coeliac disease, inflammatory bowel disease.
(4) **Poor metabolism of food:** metabolic (hypothyroidism, GH deficiency), inborn errors of metabolism (glycogen storage disorders, galactosaemia).
(5) ↑**Metabolism:** CHD, CF.
(6) **Chronic disease:** anaemia, recurrent UTIs, CRF, HIV.
(7) **Chromosomal abnormalities:** Down syndrome, Turner syndrome.

A/R: Poor socio-economic circumstances, parents with psychiatric illness.

E: Between 6 weeks to 1 year prevalence is mild in 5% and severe in 1%.

H: **General:** antenatal history, perinatal/postnatal complications, birth weight.
Feeding history: record of food consumption, e.g. frequency of breastfeeding or meals/day + snacks, frequency of bowel motions.
Social history: assess parenting skills and any possibility of neglect or abuse.

E: **General:** observe child's demeanour, level of activity, interaction with parent and sibling.
Measure: height, weight, head circumference (restriction is a late sign) and plot serially on a standard growth chart.
Signs of malnutrition: wasting, muscle loss (especially buttocks, particularly in coeliac disease).
Developmental assessment: milestones, school performance, sexual development.

P: See **A**.

I: **Bloods:** Hb, TFTs, U&E, CRP, ESR, coeliac screen (if indicated).
Specific tests: may be indicated if an organic cause is suspected, e.g. sweat test in CF, karyotype, USS renal tract.

M: **Nutritional cause:** can be treated with a balanced diet of proteins, carbohydrates, vitamins, minerals, and parental education.
Functional cause: a multidisciplinary approach is required, with involvement of social workers, GP, teachers and psychologists.
Organic cause: treat the underlying disorder.
Hospitalisation may be required for assessment and observation of feeding and behavioural patterns.

C: Developmental delay, stunting of growth, complications of underlying condition, psychological implications.

P: Depends on the duration before effective treatment begins. The longer the delay in diagnosis the less likely that normal growth and development will be achieved.

Febrile seizures

D: A seizure in the presence of fever in a child aged 6 months to 6 years with an intact CNS.

A: **Genetic:** polygenic, > 50% concordance rate in monozygotic twins.

A/R: Family history (1st or 2nd degree relative) of febrile seizures, developmental delay.

E: Affects 3–4% in W. Europe and USA, and up to 9% in Japan.
Peak age: 18 months, range (6 months to 6 years).

H: **Simple febrile seizure:** isolated, brief, generalised clonic/tonic-clonic seizures.
Complex febrile seizure: focal (clonic) movements of one limb or limbs on one side, occurs more than once during the illness or is prolonged (> 10 min).
Febrile status epilepticus: seizure of duration > 30 min (up tp 5 % of febrile seizures present as status epilepticus).

E: Febrile seizures occur in neurologically and developmentally healthy children by definition.
Exclude signs of CNS infection:
Meningitis: strongly consider if < 12 months as signs of photophobia/neck stiffness are minimal or absent.
Encephalitis: persistent drowsiness/irritability.

P: Induction of epileptiform activity by rapid rise in body temperature.

I: **LP:** if suspicion of meningitis, contraindicated with focal neurology or signs of raised ICP.
Bloods: U&Es to exclude electrolyte imbalance, WCC/CRP/blood cultures if meningitis suspected.

M: **Termination of seizure:** majority require no medical intervention. Seizures last 3–4 min. Rectal antipyretics (paracetamol, *not aspirin*) and diazepam may be used if seizure persists longer than this.
Status epilepticus requires full protocol (see Appendix).
Prophylaxis: antipyretics, diazepam (oral or rectal) at onset of febrile illness reduces probability of febrile seizure; indicated if child has a history of, or is at high risk for, prolonged or multiple seizures. Regular anti-epileptics are rarely indicated.
Reassurance and education: prevent accidental injury from fall during seizure, do not restrain. Inform of excellent prognosis with very minimal risk of epilepsy and no evidence that anti-epileptics prevent development of epilepsy.

C: **Mesial–temporal sclerosis:** associated with prolonged febrile status epilepticus (> 90 min). Results in complex partial seizures starting after a seizure-free period of variable duration. 30% of patients with mesial–temporal lobe sclerosis can be controlled with medical treatment.

P: **Recurrence:** $\frac{1}{3}$ of children will experience a recurrence. The higher the temperature at which the seizure occurred and the longer the duration of fever prior to the seizure, the lower the risk of recurrence.
Developmental sequelae: no subsequent deficit in cognitive ability/school performance.
Epilepsy: 1–2% will develop epilepsy; there is ↑risk with family history of epilepsy, neurodevelopmental abnormality, occurrence of a complex febrile seizure and shorter duration of fever prior to febrile seizure.
Mortality: is low even in febrile status epilepticus.

D: Disruption in the integrity of bone associated with soft tissue injury.

A: **Trauma:** force applied to bone exceeds its strength. The force can be direct (penetrative, crushing) or indirect (tension, compression, or rotation injuries).
Greenstick fractures: partial fracture across shaft of bone due to stronger fibrous periosteum in children.
Pathological fracture: minor force causes fracture due to underlying weakness of bone (malignancy, congenital).

A/R: Participation in contact sports, rickets, osteogenesis imperfecta.

E: **Annual UK incidence:** 36/1000 children. M > F. Incidence ↑ with age. Sports and leisure activities account for most fractures, followed by assault and then RTAs.

H: Determine mechanism of fracture and situation in which it occurred (how, where, time elapsed since injury, force experienced, possibility of glass injury), associated head injury, medications, previous injury or fractures, and a careful social history.

E: **Closed fracture:** pallor and swelling over fracture site, obvious deformity.
Open fracture: bleeding and bruising over fracture, associated soft tissue injury.
Neurovascular status: assess for distal numbness, tingling, paralysis, or loss of pulse.
Musculoskeletal: examine joint above and below for crepitus, effusion, and pain.
Tuning fork test: exacerbates pain over small stress fractures.

P: Healing of fractures involves inflammation, followed by granulation tissue formation. Chondroblasts and osteoblasts form in the granulation tissue which → callus formation. Finally lamellar bone replaces meshlike callus and is remodelled by osteoclasts.

I: **X-ray:** rule of twos; 2 views (frontal/lateral), 2 joints. Repeat 7–14 days later in fracture clinic if fracture not immediately apparent.
MRI: may be required to assess ligamentous/soft tissue injury.
Bone scan: occasionally required to exclude stress fractures.
Skeletal survey: in children with suspicion of NAI.

M: ABC protocol. Adequate analgesia. Stabilise fractures with splints.
Closed reduction: manual manipulation with adequate analgesia.
Open reduction and internal fixation: aims to adequately expose area surgically before reducing fracture using wires, plates, screws, or nails.
External fixation: avoids soft tissues that are adjacent to the fracture.
Immobilisation: with plaster casts, braces, or splints attached from joint above to joint below to allow healing. Traction by application of tension aligns ends of fracture.
Rehabilitation: important to prevent contractures and loss of function.

C: **Short-term:** neurovascular damage, malunion, non-union, delayed union of the fracture, infection (cellulitis/osteomyelitis), thromboembolic events (DVT, PE), avascular necrosis (scaphoid, femur), psychological impact of disabling condition.
Medium-term: compartment syndrome (tissue pressure rises above perfusion pressure in a closed space, e.g. cast → tissue necrosis).
Long-term: fractures involving the growth plate (Salter–Harris classification) may arrest growth. Fractures involving joint surfaces may → arthritis.

P: Typically upper limb fractures require 3–4 weeks and lower limb 6–8 weeks to heal (depends on site of fracture and health of child).

Fragile-X syndrome

D: 2nd most common form of inherited learning disability (after Down syndrome).

A: X-linked disorder with defect at distal end of long arm of X chromosome which appears 'fragile'. FMR1 gene contains CGG repeats. Extent of clinical involvement appears to correlate with length of abnormal CGG repeat sequence:
(1) **Normal:** 5–50 repeats.
(2) **Pre-mutation:** 50–230 repeats (no clinical syndrome).
(3) **Full mutation:** > 230 repeats (risk of severe neuropsychiatric disability).
Repeat sequences only increase in size when inherited through the mother.
50% of females with full mutation are phenotypically normal as they possess 2 X chromosomes.

E: 1/4000 male and 1/8000 female live births.

A/R: **Comorbidity:** Autistic spectrum disorder (15–20%), ADHD (33%), psychiatric comorbidity; schizotypal personality, depression, self-harm (up to 60% in males).
Physical: epilepsy (20%), MVP.

H: **Intellectual function:** borderline IQ that declines at around 10–15 years. Females have higher IQ.
Speech and language:

- Delayed with deficits in receptive and expressive language skills.
- Compulsive utterances and shifts in speech pitch and rate are common.
- Poor topic maintenance and tangential comments.

E: **General:** large and prominent ears, narrow facies, strabismus, macro-orchidism (only in minority of pre-pubertal males), gaze aversion on meeting in nearly all > 8 years of age.
Joint disorder: hyper-extensibility, pes planus, pectus excavatum, joint laxity, and dislocation.

P: Expansion of an unstable (CGG)n in the FMR1 gene → extensive local methylation and transcription silencing, resulting in the loss of FMRP and the development of the clinical features of fragile-X syndrome. Behavioural and cognitive features are attributed to disruption in the development of dendrites and synapses, the targets for axonal growth in the frontostriatal pathways and parietal sensory–motor tracts of the CNS.

I: **DNA testing:** to assess number of CGG triplet repeats. **EEG:** Up to 50% may have diffusely abnormal EEG although seizures only occur in about 20%.
Echo: to rule out MVP. **Spinal X-ray:** to exclude scoliosis.
MRI brain: may show ↓cerebellar vermis with ↑4th ventricular size.
Prenatal screening for fragile-X: recent studies have shown that PCR technique can be used on maternal blood samples from 8 weeks gestation with 99% detection rate.

M: **Multidisciplinary team approach:**
Educational input: training for memory and reading, may need to attend school for children with special needs.
Speech and language therapy.
Orthopaedic referral: for gait dyspraxia and scoliosis.
Treatment of comorbidity: methylphenidate (ADHD), antidepressants, anxiolytics.
Folate supplementation: benefits of supplementation are equivocal.

C: Scoliosis, loss of visual acuity.

P: Normal life expectancy; however, condition can be very disabling due to comorbidity and extent of learning disability.

Ringworm

D: **Dermatophytosis (fungal infection) of keratin layer of skin, nails, or hair.**
Called *ringworm* due to annular skin lesions produced.

A: Dermatophyte fungi infect the skin, nails, or hair, reproduce by spore formation, and induce inflammation by delayed hypersensitivity or metabolic effects.
3 genera of fungi responsible:
(1) *Microsporum* (infect skin and hair).
(2) *Trichophyton* (infect skin, nail, and hair).
(3) *Epidermophyton* (infect skin and nail).
Infections include: tinea capitis (scalp), tinea pedis (feet = athlete's foot), tinea unguium (nails), tinea corporis (trunk and limbs), tinea cruris (groin). (Tinea = latin for worm.)

A/R: Humid, sweaty conditions, e.g. occlusive footwear, moist body folds, hyperhidrosis. Topical steroid use. Tinea capitis is often acquired from cats and dogs.

E: Tinea capitis is more common in children of African descent in whom scalp and hair are more susceptible to fungal infection.

H: Generally itchy, red patches. In tinea capitis, hairs break just above the scalp, producing a *black dot* appearance.

E: Depends on infection; generally ringworm occurs as asymmetrical, scaly, erythematous annular patches with an advancing raised border, central clearing and occasional vesicles/pustules at edge. In tinea capitis patchy alopecia occurs. In tinea pedis typical annular lesions are rarely seen, usually skin in toe clefts is white and fissured.

P: Diagnosis is clinical, therefore rarely biopsied. Dermatophytes infect keratin as branching hyphae. Silver stains and neutral polysaccharides stains (PAS) react with cell walls and reveal dermatophytes.

I: **Wood's light:** some fungi fluoresce greenish/yellow under Wood's light (filtered UV light).
Microscopy: skin scrapings placed on a slide with 10% aqueous potassium hydroxide to examine for hyphae. Gives almost immediate diagnosis.
Culture: skin scrapings, nail clippings, or hair may be cultured in a medium for 3 weeks to identify the fungus.

M: **Topical antifungals:** imidazoles (canesten) for tinea pedis and localised skin lesions.
Systemic antifungals: griseofulvin for scalp and nail infections and for widespread lesions.

C: Kerion formation; severe inflammatory, pustular scalp ringworm patch.

P: Resolves with appropriate treatment.

Pityriasis versicolor

D: Chronic, asymptomatic, fungal infection characterised by pigmentary changes on the trunk.

A: Overgrowth of commensal yeast *Pityrosporum orbiculare (Malassezia furfur).*

A/R: Humid tropical conditions.

E: Commonest yeast infection in adolescence.

H: Asymptomatic rash on trunk and upper arms.

E: Caucasians: reddish brown scaly macules.
Black-skinned patients: macular areas of hypopigmentation.

P: Microscopic: 'grapes and bananas' appearance of spores and short hyphae.

I: Skin scrapings for microscopy and culture, fluorescence by Wood's light.

M: Selenium sulphide shampoo/topical imidazoles/oral itraconazole.

C: Inappropriate topical steroids spread the rash.

P: Pigmentation takes months to recover. Recurrences are common.

D: Inflammation of the GI tract 2° to acute infection.

A: **Viruses:** rotavirus (commonest), adeno, calici, corona, and astroviruses.
Bacteria:
(1) **Neurotoxin-producing:** *Staphylococcus aureus* and *Bacillus cereus*; cause severe vomiting shortly after ingestion, rarely cause diarrhoea.
(2) **Enterotoxin-producing:** *Escherichia coli* and *Vibrio cholerae* act directly on secretory mechanisms primarily by ↑activation of cAMP and produce typically copious watery diarrhoea (rice water). No mucosal invasion occurs.
(3) **Cytotoxin-producing:** *Shigella dysenteriae, Vibrio parahaemolyticus, Clostridium difficile,* and enterohaemorrhagic *E. coli* result in mucosal cell destruction → bloody stools with inflammatory cells.
(4) **Mucosal invasion:** *Shigella, Campylobacter,* and enteroinvasive *E. coli* cause mucosal destruction and inflammatory diarrhoea. *Salmonella* and *Yersinia* species also invade cells but do not cause cell death. Hence, dysentery does not usually occur. These bacteria will, however, invade the blood stream across the lamina propria and cause enteric fever such as typhoid.

A/R: Poverty, malnutrition, lack of infrastructure, bottle-feeding, antibiotic use, and immunocompromise.

E: **Worldwide:** 3–5 billion cases/year.
UK: average child experiences 2 episodes of diarrhoea/year.

H: **General:** fever, anorexia, vomiting, abdominal pain, and diarrhoea.
Specific: features of diarrhoea and time lapse in between ingestion of food and symptoms may suggest infective organism (see **A**).

E: Assess degree of dehydration by loss of body weight in %.
Mild (< 5%): no clinical signs.
Moderate (> 5%): dry mucous membranes, ↓skin turgor, cool peripheries.
Severe (10%): skin laxity, sunken eyes and fontanelle, impaired peripheral circulation, acidotic breathing, restlessness, lethargy, and oliguria.
Extreme (10–15%): anuria, shock, or coma.

P: Dehydration is the result of impaired absorption of water, electrolytes, and sugars following mucosal damage or ↑ in secretory mechanisms.

I: **General:** weight and temperature monitoring.
Bloods: FBC, U&E, LFTs. **Stool:** microscopy, culture and sensitivity.

M: **Mild dehydration:** short-term substitution of normal feeds with maintenance-type of oral glucose–electrolyte solution (Diarolyte), until the vomiting and profuse diarrhoea subside.
Moderate dehydration: 6-h trial of oral rehydration (PO or NG if not tolerating fluids) with 100 ml/kg/24h. If no improvement, IV rehydration should be administered.
Severe dehydration: IV rehydration. Treat shocked patients with plasma expanders. Fluid deficit replacement should be given as well as maintenance fluid requirement and allowances for future losses. Potassium supplementation should commence once the patient is passing urine.
ORT: in the developing world this simple, inexpensive, glucose–electrolyte solution promoted by the WHO has reduced the number of deaths from dehydration due to diarrhoea by about a million/year.

C: Dehydration, post-gastroenteritis syndrome, ARF in severe dehydration.

P: **Developing countries:** 5 million children <5 years die/year.
Developed countries: 1% mortality.

Gastrointestinal (GI) atresia

D: Congenital malformation of the GI tract resulting in a blind pouch and obstruction.

A: The commonest sites for atresia are the oesophagus, the duodenum, and the anus. The frequent association with other congenital anomalies points to a developmental rather than an acquired origin.

Oesophageal atresia: In 85% there is a blind proximal oesophageal pouch with a distal oesophageal to tracheal fistula. In 10% there is oesophageal atresia without a fistula. In 5% there is proximal (H-type) fistula +/- distal fistula without oesophageal atresia.

Duodenal atresia: the duodenum ends in a blind pouch distal to the ampulla of Vater in 75% of cases and proximal in 25% of cases. The atresia may be continuous with the bowel wall, may be joined with a fibrous cord to the normal bowel, or may be completely separate.

Anal atresia: the rectum either ends in a blind pouch without connection to the colon, or opens onto the urethra, bladder or scrotum in boys and vagina in girls.

A/R: **Oesophageal:** 50% of patients with TOF have VACTERL anomalies and other midline defects (cleft palate defects, sacral dysgenesis, urogenital anomalies), maternal polyhydramnios, Down syndrome.

Duodenal: maternal polyhydramnios, Down syndrome, congenital cardiac abnormalities, malrotation, early intrauterine intussusception.

Anal: affected sibling, oesophageal, urinary tract, and bone abnormalities, VACTERL anomalies.

E: **Oesophageal:** 1/3500 live births.
Duodenal: 1/5000 live births.
Anal: 1/5000 live births.

H: The presence of polyhydramnios in the mother during the last trimester of pregnancy should alert the doctor to the possibility of a high intestinal obstruction.

Oesophageal: at birth the infant is unable to swallow saliva and presents with froth at the mouth. Aspiration of saliva causes choking attacks, cyanotic episodes and may produce pneumonia affecting the right upper or middle lobes.

Duodenal: persistent bilious vomiting or clear vomitus if the defect is proximal (supra-ampullary), passage of little or no meconium in 50%.

Anal: usually detected during routine examination, if not will present later with intestinal obstruction.

E: **Oesophageal:** abdominal distension with an associated fistula, or 'scaphoid' (sunken/nondistended) abdomen if there is no fistula.

Duodenal: may present with upper abdominal distension.

Anal: absence of the anal margins and inability to pass a small-gauge NG tube.

P: See **A**.

I: **Oesophageal:** diagnosis is confirmed by passing a large-calibre radio-opaque catheter into the oesophagus. An erect CXR will determine the level of the atresia as the catheter will fail to reach the stomach and will be coiled in the pouch. The presence of gas in the stomach is indicative of a distal TOF. Contrast studies are potentially dangerous as spillover into the trachea may occur.

Duodenal: AXR shows a dilated proximal bowel (double bubble sign) and absent or reduced gas beyond the obstruction. Fluid levels are common. Barium enemas may help distinguish duodenal atresia from other pathologies such as a meconium ileus.

Anal: AXR shows the defect when the colon is enhanced with contrast. May also be identified on USS.

M: Early surgical intervention is necessary as there is usually complete intestinal obstruction.

Oesophageal: immediate transfer to a neonatal surgical centre. During transfer the neonate should be placed head-up and prone in order to prevent the regurgitation of gastric contents into the trachea via a TOF if present. Suction should be applied to the oesophageal pouch. Keep NBM. Surgical repair depends on the oesophageal length; may be achieved by 1° end-to-end anastomosis or a staged repair with a feeding gastrostomy and defunctioning cervical oesophagostomy followed by a colonic transplant.

Duodenal: pre-op correction of fluid and electrolyte abnormalities. Gastric decompression by NG tube insertion. Surgical bypass of the defect, or direct end-to-end anastomosis is usually achieved after limited resection.

Anal: anal dilatation may be needed in a narrowed anus. Initially a defunctioning colostomy is performed. Subsequently a functioning rectum is achieved via perineal anoplasty. The colostomy is reversed a few months after this.

C: Aspiration pneumonia, NEC.

P: Mortality is directly related to the severity of the associated anomalies and to the degree of prematurity. Overall mortality rate in oesophageal atresia is 20% and in duodenal atresia 20–30%. Mortality in anal atresia is low.

Gastro-oesophageal reflux disease (GORD)

D: ↑Movement of gastric contents from the stomach into the oesophagus.

A: **GOR:** normal in infants, predisposing factors are:
(1) Supine position.
(2) Short, straight intra-abdominal length of the oesophagus.
(3) Immature, relaxed gastro-oesophageal sphincter.
GORD: occurs when reflux frequency and duration produce symptoms. Common mechanisms:
(1) Delay in neurological maturation (e.g. preterm infants).
(2) Neurological impairment (cerebral palsy, HIE, Down syndrome).
(3) Excessive frequent spontaneous reductions in sphincter pressure (crying, coughing, or defaecation).

A/R: Cow's milk protein intolerance.

E: **Prevalence:** 1/3000 infants. GORD is often overdiagnosed and therefore overtreated.

H&E: There is a wide range of clinical presentation for GORD, ranging from mild irritation to severe disease. Symptoms can involve both the GI system as well as the respiratory system, especially if there are associated neurological problems or anatomical abnormalities (cleft palate, TOF).
General: avoidance of feeding (associating with discomfort), or constant eating/drinking (milk is antacid and therefore relieves symptoms), irritability (discomfort of acid indigestion), arching of back.
GI: difficulty/pain on swallowing, vomiting after feeds, haematemesis, gastric/abdominal/retrosternal pain.
Respiratory: apnoea, intermittent stridor, recurrent pneumonia.

P: See **A**.

I: **24-h pH monitoring of the oesophagus:** gold standard for diagnosis; however, needs careful interpretation as GOR is normal and may reduce the pH of the oesophagus.
Impedance testing: more sensitive technique in testing small changes in pH levels in the oesophagus by measuring resistance to electrical currents within the lining of the oesophagus.
Contrast studies: upper GI tract to exclude anatomical abnormalities.
Endoscopy: due to the episodic nature of GORD ~50% of patients with severe symptoms will have no endoscopic findings, so only do if oesophagitis is suspected.

M: **Conservative:** time and reassurance unless child is exhibiting failure to thrive. Thicken feeds, ↓volume and ↑frequency of feeds, position infant upright for 30 min after feeding.
Pharmacological: H_2-antagonists or proton pump inhibitors are used only in severe GORD or if oesophagitis has been shown on endoscopy.
Laparoscopic Nissen fundoplication: creates a valve at the top of the stomach by wrapping a portion of the stomach around the oesophagus. May be necessary for severe, intractable symptoms that are usually in association with neurological impairment.

C: **General:** failure to thrive, Sandifer syndrome (dystonic movements of the head and neck). **GI:** oesophagitis, peptic stricture.
Respiratory: pulmonary aspiration due to neurological immaturity may → pneumonia and apnoea in preterm infants.

P: Majority of GORD resolves by 1 year. This is probably due to the maturation of the lower oesophageal sphincter.

D: Genetic disorders of skeletal development and growth, which can be divided into the chondrodysplasias (e.g. achondroplasia) and the osteodysplasias (e.g. osteogenesis imperfecta).

A: **Chondrodysplasia:** mutations in genes for cartilage matrix proteins, transmembrane receptors, transcription factors, and ion transporters.

- **Achondroplasia:** autosomal dominant condition involving mutation in the FGFR3 gene on chromosome 4 (50% *de novo* mutations).

Osteodysplasia: mutations in genes → abnormal development of bone.

- **Osteogenesis imperfecta (brittle bone disease):** autosomal dominant mutations that code for Type I procollagen.

A/R: Achondroplasia is associated with higher paternal age.

E: **Achondroplasia: incidence:** 0.5–1.5/10 000/year.
Osteogenesis imperfecta: incidence: 1/20 000/year.

H&E: **Achondroplasia:** average trunk length with shortened limbs, megalocephaly, short stature, and angular deformities of the extremities. Cervicomedullary compression may present with ataxia, pain, apnoea, or incontinence.
Osteogenesis imperfecta:
Type I (mild): recurrent childhood fractures, blue sclera, early deafness.
Type II (most severe): may be stillborn or die in infancy from respiratory insufficiency. Extreme fragility, low birth weight, and small thorax.
Type III: *in utero* fractures, macrocephaly, triangular facies, scoliosis, and vertebral compression.
Type IV: moderate short stature and bowing of legs; sustain fractures but are often mobile in the community.

P: **Achondroplasia:** ↑function of the FGFR3 gene → reduced endochondrial ossification.
Osteogenesis imperfecta: in normal bone formation, Type I collagen contains 3 chains composed of uninterrupted repeats of Glycine-X-Y. In osteogenesis imperfecta, the matrix of bone is composed of abnormal Type I collagen caused by substitution of glycine by other residues.

I: **Achondroplasia:**
Radiology: large skull cap bones, small cranial base and facial bones.
MRI cervical spine: for cervical stenosis.
Osteogenesis imperfecta:
DEXA scan: bone mass density is ~75% of normal.
Lumbar spine X-rays: for compression fractures.
Collagen synthesis analysis.

M: **Achondroplasia:** GH/insulin-like growth factor, neurological follow-up, surgical decompression of cervical stenosis, leg-lengthening procedures.
Osteogenesis imperfecta: prompt fracture splinting or casting and correction of deformity to restore function, physiotherapy in younger children, mobility aids (braces, wheelchairs).

C: **Achondroplasia:** craniocervical stenosis may → spinal cord compression, subsequent quadriparesis and respiratory arrest.
Osteogenesis imperfecta: recurrent pneumonia, brainstem compression, hydrocephalus, and syringohydromyelia.

P: **Achondroplasia:** individuals have normal lifespan and intelligence.
Osteogenesis imperfecta:

- *Type I* and *IV* are associated with a normal lifespan.
- *Type III* are susceptible to respiratory problems and have a ↓lifespan.
- *Type II* usually die in infancy.

Global developmental delay

D: Delay in acquisition of all developmental milestones, particularly language, fine motor, and social skills. Usually indicates learning disability.

A: **Genetic:** chromosomal abnormalities (Down syndrome, fragile-X syndrome), inborn errors of metabolism.
Environmental: emotional deprivation, neglect, NAI.
Intrauterine: infections (TORCH), toxins (alcohol, anticonvulsants).
Perinatal: asphyxia, birth trauma, instrumental delivery, hypoglycaemia (prolonged).
Postnatal: meningitis, encephalitis, head trauma, uncontrolled seizures.
Metabolic: congenital hypothyroidism, lead poisoning.
CNS abnormalities: hydrocephalus, neural tube defects.
Neurodegenerative: cerebral palsy, mucopolysaccharidoses, lysozomal and lipid storage disorders.
Neurocutaneous: NF, TS.
Neuromuscular: DMD/BMD, myotonic dystrophy.
Idiopathic: autistic spectrum disorder.

A/R: Family history of learning disability or consanguinity, epilepsy, ADHD, impairment of vision and hearing, communication deficits.

E: **Severe learning disability (IQ $<$ 50):** 4/1000 children.
Moderate learning disability (IQ 50–69): 20/1000 children.

H: **Child's current skills; previous milestones; regression in skills.**
History of pregnancy/delivery: alcohol, drugs, mode and complications of delivery, birth weight, length, and head circumference.
Postnatal complications: hypoglycaemia, jaundice, apnoea, feeding difficulties, failure to thrive, admission to SCBU.
Previous illness: meningitis, encephalitis, head injury.
A careful social history.

E: Measure current weight, length, and head circumference, and plot on growth centile chart. Examine for dysmorphic features, neurological abnormalities (assess muscle tone, strength, coordination, cranial nerves, primitive reflexes), assess vision, hearing and development, perform general physical examination (e.g. for pigmentation, hepatosplenomegaly), look for signs of neglect or abuse.

P: See **A**.

I: **Depends on history and examination:**
Bloods: TFTs, mucopolysaccharide screening, serology for congenital infections, creatine phosphokinase.
Karyotype: including DNA testing for fragile-X syndrome.
Cranial imaging: MRI/CT.
Other: EEG if having seizures, urine metabolic screening.

M: **Multidisciplinary approach:**
Determine cause: important for genetic advice and because some causes are treatable (hypothyroidism).
Parental and sibling support: education, genetic counselling, and emotional support.
Assessment of needs: learning ability, mobility (physiotherapy), and safety (crossing roads).
Educational programmes: early intervention to stimulate cognitive, language, and motor development. Adaptive techniques in visually/hearing impaired.
Statement of special educational needs: notify education authority to ensure needs are met.

Behaviour management: mild; ADHD, moderate to severe; stereotypical, self-injurious behaviour.
Paediatric care: under specialist where appropriate (neurodegenerative, neuromuscular, neurocutaneous).

C: Psychological problems in 50%, behavioural problems in 30%, dependent lifestyle.

P: ↑Mortality especially in early childhood due to respiratory infections, seizures, and associated congenital anomalies (e.g. CHD in Down syndrome).
Degree of independent living depends on degree of learning disability and underlying aetiology.
Mild to moderate learning disability: may achieve independent lifestyle in sheltered accommodation and workshops or in local authority occupation centres.
Severe learning disability: require constant supervision by family and later in residential homes.

Glomerulonephritis (GN), acute

D: Characterised by the appearance of blood and protein in the urine in association with ↓ GFR, oliguria, oedema, and hypertension.

A: **Post-streptococcal:** 2° to group A β-haemolytic streptococcal infection.
HUS: haemolytic anaemia, thrombocytopaenia, and endothelial damage to the glomerular capillaries 2° to infection by *E.coli* 0157, *Shigella*, or *Salmonella*.
HSP: hypersensitivity vasculitis and inflammatory response within the glomerular capillaries with associated petechiae, rash, abdominal pain, and arthritis.
IgA nephropathy: deposits of IgA antibodies in the renal mesangial tissue.
SLE nephritis: the immune system produces antinuclear antibodies. Complexes of these antibodies and complement accumulate in the kidneys and result in an inflammatory response.

A/R: Preceding sore throat/impetigo (post-streptococcal GN), URTI (HSP), or GI infection (HUS).

E: **Post-streptococcal:** 1/13 000; peak age 6–10 years; peak presentation is during the winter months, less common now because of antibiotic use.
HUS: 1/10 000; peak age 3 months to 3 years.
HSP: peak age 3–10 years, M : F = 2 : 1.
IgA nephropathy: most commonly affects males in their teens.
SLE: uncommon in children. F > M.

H: Haematuria, oliguria, swelling of face, ankles, abdomen (ascites), symptoms of ↑BP (nose bleeds, headache), malaise, fever, anorexia, abdominal pain, preceding URTI (HSP), preceding gastroenteritis (HUS).

E: Petechiae; buttock and extensor surface (HSP), measure BP.

P: Immunologically mediated glomerular injury by antigen–antibody-immune complexes trapped in the renal parenchyma. A process of inflammation and cell proliferation is initiated, which damages normal renal tissue.

I: **Urine:** microscopy to detect RBC +/− casts and culture, 24-h collection; protein and creatinine clearance.
Bloods: ↓Hb, ↑WCC, ↓Plt (HUS), ↑urea, ↑ESR/CRP, metabolic acidosis.
Determine aetiology:
Post-streptococcal: throat swab, ASOT, ↓ C_3, normal C_4 complement level.
HUS: RBC fragmentation, stool culture.
HSP: usually clinical diagnosis.
IgA: ↑IgA antibodies.
SLE: ANA, persistently ↓C_3 complement levels.
Imaging: renal USS.
Renal biopsy: for definitive diagnosis; not usually required.

M: **Supportive:** salt and protein restriction, monitor BP and treat if >140/100 with frusemide. Renal dialysis may be indicated in severe cases (HUS).
Post-streptococcal: penicillin to destroy remaining streptococcal infection.
HUS/SLE: steroids and/or immunosuppressants.

C: **Hypertension:** encephalopathy, convulsions, end-organ damage, cerebral haemorrhage.
Renal failure: uraemia, metabolic acidosis, electrolyte abnormalities, fluid overload.

P: **Post-streptococcal:** good for >90%; acute phase lasts 1–2 weeks, hypertension for 3–4 weeks, and microscopic haematuria for up to 12 months, but rapidly progressive to CRF in 1%.
HUS: a life-threatening condition; mortality 5–30%, some may relapse.
IgA nephropathy: 10–30% progress to CRF.
HSP: usually resolves spontaneously without treatment, 1–2% develop CRF.
SLE nephritis: condition may change its severity over time.

D: Bacterial infection caused by *Streptococcus agalactiae*, which is a gram-positive Group B β-haemolytic streptococcus that causes invasive disease in pregnant women and their newborn infants.

A: GBS is a common infection in the adult population. Infection can be subclinical; therefore many patients are carriers; it colonises the colon, vagina, bladder, or throat. A foetus is at maximum risk if the maternal infection is either colonic or vaginal in origin, and transmission can occur either in the antenatal, perinatal, or postnatal period.
There are 2 forms of infection:
Early:
- Occurs in infants $<1/52$ old.
- Acquired through vertical transmission from colonised mothers.
- Commonly presents with sepsis, pneumonia, and/or meningitis.

Late:
- Occurs in infants $>1/52$ old.
- Acquired by either vertical transmission (delayed infection after early colonisation) or by horizontal infection (in the hospital or community).
- Meningitis is the most common presentation (85%).

A/R: Preterm labour ($<37/40$), prolonged rupture of membranes (>18 h in preterm infants, >24 h in term infants), maternal fever, GBS bacteriuria during pregnancy, chorioamnionitis, previous delivery of a GBS neonate (regardless of current maternal colonisation status).

E: 20–30% of pregnant women are colonised with GBS; neonatal incidence is typically 1–5/1000 live births/yr. With heavy maternal colonisation this rises to 1/25 of all live births. Late onset is less common.

H&E: **Sepsis:** temperature instability (fever, hypothermia) hypo/hyperglycaemia, irritability, drowsiness, lethargy, seizures, poor feeding, vomiting, jaundice, abdominal distension, respiratory distress, apnoea, bradycardia or shock.
Meningitis: as for sepsis with tense or bulging fontanelle and head retraction (opisthotonos).
Pneumonia: usually presents with respiratory distress; tachypnoea, recession, nasal flaring, expiratory grunting, tachycardia, and cyanosis (severe cases).

P: See **A**.

I: **Full septic screen:**
Bloods: ↑WCC, ↑/↓ glucose, ↑CRP, U&E, LFTs.
Culture: blood, urine, CSF (LP).
Radiology: CXR.

M: **Prevention:**
- Identification of at-risk infants (See **A**).
- Culture from the vaginal introitus and anorectum in mothers with at-risk features.
- Intrapartum IV benzyl-penicillin (clindamycin if allergic) should be used >4 h prior to delivery.

Treatment:
- Broad-spectrum antibiotics should be started immediately before receiving results of cultures.
- Includes IV benzyl-penicillin and gentamycin (which act synergistically against GBS), or ampicillin and gentamycin as ampicillin gives additional cover against Listeria.
- Serial CRP measurements may help to monitor response.

C: Hearing and visual impairment, developmental delay.

P: Morbidity is 5% in neonates although neonatal meningitis has a mortality of 20–50%.

Haemophilia, A and B

D: Bleeding diatheses resulting from inherited deficiency of a clotting factor. **HA:** FVIII deficiency, **HB:** FIX deficiency.

A: X-linked recessive conditions. 30% of cases arise due to de novo mutation.

A/R: Family history, males with carrier mothers, consanguinity.

E: **HA:** 1/10 000 males. **HB:** 1/50 000 males.

H: Severity of disease and its presentation is proportional to the level and therefore activity of the clotting factor.
Severe (< 1% activity):
(1) Neonates after circumcision.
(2) < 1 year old: bruising (may present as ?NAI).
(3) Toddlers: deep muscle bleeds and haemarthroses by 3 years, oral and gum bleeding from minor lacerations and losing teeth.
(4) Older children: joint deformity and ankylosis.
Moderate (1–5% activity): bleeding after mild–moderate trauma, few spontaneous bleeds.
Mild (5–25% activity): bleeding after moderate–severe trauma, or surgery.

E: Multiple bruises, muscle haematomas, haemarthroses, joint deformities which → limited range of movement, nerve palsies.

P: **HA:** FVIII is a vital cofactor in the intrinsic pathway of the coagulation cascade. When activated by thrombin, it accelerates the activity of the clotting cascade 200 000-fold.
HB: activated FIX (FIXa) converts FX to FXa in the intrinsic pathway.
Deficiency of either FVIII or FIX therefore gives rise to an ↑time for clot formation, i.e. bleeding diatheses. This results in a prolonged APTT, which reflects the activity of the intrinsic and the final common pathway.

I: **Coagulation studies:** ↑APTT.
Coagulation factor assays: ↓FVIII (HA), ↓FIX (HB).
Genetic studies: karyotype analysis of patient and family.
Other investigations according to complications, e.g. arthroscopy.

M: **Regular follow-up at a haemophilia centre.**
Mild bleeding:
(1) Desmopressin (vasopressin analogue) intranasally/IV mobilises FVIII from stores.
(2) Tranexamic acid (contraindicated in haematuria).
(3) FVIII (HA)/FIX (HB) concentrate infusions.
Maintain levels to 20–50% of normal when treating active bleeding.
Severe bleeding/surgery: FVIII (HA)/FIX (HB) IV concentrate infusions. Maintain levels to 70–100% of normal until resolution. 10–15% of patients develop antibodies to the clotting factor particularly recipients of FVIII. This requires specialised haematological management.
Education: avoid antiplatelet drugs (aspirin), IM injections, contact sports; provide genetic counselling.
Immunisations: hepatitis A and B.
Specialist referral for complications: orthopaedic.
Medic alert card/bracelet.

C: Severe/fatal haemorrhage, crippling joint deformity, cerebrovascular accidents, HCV and HIV infection in patients who received clotting concentrates before 1985 in developed countries, and even today in developing countries.

P: Virally screened blood products and home treatment programmes; home-administered prophylactic therapy 2–3×/week, means that most patients with haemophilia can now lead a relatively normal life.

D: Infestation of the head with lice.

A: **Pediculus humanus capitis:** 6-legged, flat, wingless, blood-sucking louse up to 3 mm long with legs adapted to cling onto hair shafts.
Mechanism of spread: head-to-head contact, sharing of hats, combs, hair-bands, and towels. Eggs (nits) can live for up to 1 month away from the body.

A/R: Young age, close crowded living conditions, warm weather.

E: **Incidence:** under-reported due to social stigma, namely the preconceived notion that lice are related to poor personal hygiene. F > M due to social acceptance of close physical contact; sharing hats, combs, hairties.
Peak age: 3–11 years 2° to close contact in classrooms and day-care facilities.
Race: Caucasians > African-Caribbeans.

H: Parents often seek assessment for their school-age children after becoming aware of an outbreak at school. Pruritus is the major complaint.

E: **Neck:** urticarial papules and/or excoriations, post-occipital +/− cervical lymphadenopathy.
Scalp: live lice on scalp and empty egg cases (nits) on hairs. The eggs are cemented firmly to the scalp hairs and appear as small white oval capsules when empty; they remain attached to the hair as it grows.

P: The bites introduce enzymes, an anticlotting agent, and a local anaesthetic into the puncture wound and produce a typical allergic reaction with concomitant itching. With repeated exposure to the bites, sensitisation occurs with an inflammatory papular dermatitis.

I: Wood's light examination reveals yellow and/or green fluorescence of the lice and their nits.

M: **Non-drug management:** solvents that help to dissolve the cement away from the nit aid in mechanical removal of nits with fine-tooth combs. In most studies that compare mechanical removal with a pediculicide, the former is not as effective.
Drug management:
(1) Pediculicides: malathion solution or permethrin cream is applied to hair overnight. After shampooing lice and nits are removed with a fine-toothed comb. This is not very effective against developing nits; therefore a 2nd treatment is required after 7 days.
(2) Co-trimoxazole p.o. has also been found to be effective.
Drug resistance: malathion and permethrin resistance is increasingly common, and rotational treatment strategies are recommended by health authorities.
Environmental eradication: pillowcases, linens, towels, toys, and hats should be washed in hot water and dried.
Treatment of contacts: treatment of family members, friends, and/or other close contacts is very important in helping to prevent further spread of lice and reinfestation.

C: **2° bacterial infection:** impetigo requires treatment and may mask underlying lice infestation.
Psychosocial impact: 2° to stigma associated with lice infestation.

P: Good with appropriate treatment, environmental eradication, and treatment of contacts.

Hearing impairment

D: **Conductive hearing loss:** sound vibrations are not conducted via the ear canal, tympanic membrane, or the ossicles. Maximum 20–60 dB hearing loss.
Sensorineural hearing loss: dysfunction of the cochlear (sensory) components or the auditory nerve. May have profound $>$ 90 dB hearing loss.

A: **Conductive hearing loss:** most cases due to secretory otitis media (glue ear).
- **Ear canal:** wax, foreign body.
- **Tympanic membrane:** perforation due to blow to ear, pressure change in aircraft.
- **Ossicles:** absent/defective ossicles due to congenital malformation.
- **Eustachian tube dysfunction:** cleft palate, Down syndrome.

Sensorineural hearing loss:
- **Genetic (50%):** autosomal recessive/dominant or as part of a syndrome, e.g. Waardenburg syndrome.
- **Intrauterine (10%):** congenital infections (rubella, CMV, herpes), aminoglycosides, loop diuretics.
- **Perinatal (10%):** birth asphyxia, preterm delivery, hyperbilirubinaemia.
- **Postnatal (30%):** measles, mumps, meningitis, encephalitis, head injury, neurodegenerative disorders.

A/R: Recurrent otitis media, URTIs, atopy.

E: **Severe:** 1/1000 children require special education (may be sensorineural or mixed).
Moderate: 2/1000 children require hearing aids and educational support.
Mild: 1/100 school-age children affected (usually 2° to glue ear and usually transient).

H: Usually suspected by mother when the baby consistently fails to respond to loud noises. May report delayed language development, behavioural or educational difficulties. Elicit family history, consanguinity, intrauterine, perinatal, or postnatal complications, recurrent otitis media or URTIs.

E: **Universal neonatal hearing screening programme:** currently being piloted in the UK. Use of otoacoustic emissions and/or auditory brainstem-evoked responses at 4–6 weeks. In this test, a computer-based system detects electrical activity in the cochlea and auditory pathways in the brain.
Distraction test ($>$4 months): infant is held on parent's lap and distracted by a toy in front. The examiner stands behind parent and creates noises of different intensities and pitches (voice, keys, rattle) to test each ear separately. Normal head-turning responses are elicited towards the side of the sound stimulus.
McCormick's toy discrimination test ($>$2 years): phonetically similar-sounding toys; duck/cup, tree/key are named and the child is asked to identify them.

P: See **A**.

I: **Impedance audiometry testing ($>$4 years):** child usually cooperates so that a quantitative pure tone threshold audiogram can be obtained for different frequencies for both air and bone conduction.

M: **Conductive hearing impairment:** assess cause and treat specifically, e.g. removal of wax.
(1) Secretory otitis media 'glue ear'; decongestants and antibiotics are ineffectual. If there is persistent hearing loss, 'grommets' (tiny plastic tubes) inserted into the tympanic membrane allow fluid to drain out and ventilate the middle ear.

(2) Myringoplasty for tympanic membrane perforation.
(3) Reconstruction for congenital ossicular chain abnormalities.

Sensorineural hearing impairment:

(1) Early diagnosis is key in implementing support mechanisms for child to achieve full potential:
- Hearing aids or cochlear implants if insufficient amplification.
- Auditory training by peripatetic teacher, who can later advise on school placement.
- Many children learn to understand the spoken word and will develop intelligible speech.
- Lip-reading and sign language are additional means of communication.

(2) Parental counselling on safety hazards, behavioural difficulties, and genetics.

C: Delayed speech and language, falling behind at school, behavioural problems.

P: **Conductive hearing impairment:** most causes are treatable or spontaneously resolve.

Sensorineural hearing impairment: good if detected early to implement necessary support and prevent educational and behavioural problems.

Heart failure

D: Heart failure: results when the heart can no longer meet the metabolic demands of the body.
CHF: refers to ↑venous pressure in the pulmonary (left heart failure) or systemic (right heart failure) veins. This occurs when the compensatory mechanisms used to improve cardiac output are no longer adequate, so heart failure becomes uncompensated.

A: In utero: severe anaemia 2° to haemolysis, arrhythmias; SVT, VT, CHB.
Preterm neonate: fluid overload, PDA, VSD, BPD.
Full-term neonate:
(1) Left heart obstruction: COA, hypoplastic left heart, aortic stenosis.
(2) Overloaded system: PDA.
(3) TGA.
(4) Pump failure (rare): viral, ischaemic, or metabolic.
(5) Arteriovenous malformation: hepatic.
Infant–toddler: VSD; left → right cardiac shunts, arteriovenous malformations, post-op repair of congenital cardiac defects.
Child–adolescent: acute hypertension (GN), viral myocarditis.

A/R: Down, Turner, Marfan, and Noonan syndromes. Drugs, chemicals, and infections.

E: Rare in children; more common in infants with CHD.

H: Infants: breathlessness, wheeze (cardiac asthma), grunting, feeding difficulties, sweating, failure to thrive, recurrent chest infections.
Older children: fatigue, exercise intolerance, dizziness, or syncope.

E: Left CHF: tachycardia, tachypnoea, signs of respiratory distress (recession), gallop rhythm, displaced apex, absence of a heart murmur does not exclude heart disease (TGA, hypoplastic left heart, COA).
Right CHF: hepatosplenomegaly and oedema or ascites. Jugular venous distension is not a reliable indicator of systemic venous congestion in infants because the jugular veins are difficult to examine.
Uncompensated CHF: hypotension, cool extremities with poor peripheral perfusion, thready pulse, and ↓urine output, signs of renal and hepatic failure in severe cases.

P: Cardiac output = stroke volume × HR.
BP = cardiac output × systemic vascular resistance (SVR).
In progressive heart failure, cardiac output drops and is initially compensated for by ↑HR, then ↑ SVR (cool peripheries). Once these are no longer sufficient there is ↓BP which is pre-terminal.

I: CXR: cardiomegaly, ↑pulmonary vascular markings and fluid collection in the pulmonary fields may be detected.
ECG: rate, rhythm, atrial and ventricular hypertrophy or hypoplasia.
Echo: diagnostic for congenital heart defects.
Cardiac catheterisation: measures intracardiac pressures and shunts/used for therapeutic purposes.

M: This is an emergency requiring admission to a specialist unit.
General: rest (↓cardiac work), oxygen, Na^+/fluid restriction.
Medical: combination of loop and thiazide diuretics. β-blockers are not beneficial in children.
Surgical: cardiogenic transplantation, external left ventricular support devices.

C: Arrhythmias, SVT, VT, CHB, cardiogenic shock.

P: Poor for severe heart failure in children with the absence of a correctable congenital cardiac lesion.

D: Congenital defect in the formation of the diaphragm that → the protrusion of abdominal contents into the thoracic cavity.

A: **General:**

- Can be unilateral or bilateral; unilateral is more common, L > R.
- In left-sided hernias small and large bowel as well as solid intra-abdominal organs herniate.
- In right-sided hernias the liver and a portion of the large bowel herniate.
- CDH is associated with a variable degree of pulmonary hypoplasia due to a decrease in the cross-sectional area of the pulmonary vasculature and dysfunction of surfactant.

Posterolateral Bochdalek's hernia:

- 90% of cases; left-sided, occurs *in utero* at ~6 weeks gestation.
- Caused by a posterolateral defect in the diaphragm, which results from the failure of the pleuroperitoneal folds to develop or the improper or absent migration of the diaphragmatic musculature.

Morgagni's hernia:

- Less common CDH (5–10% of cases), 90% are right-sided.
- Anterior midline defect through the sternocostal hiatus of the diaphragm.

Congenital hiatus hernia:

- Very rare in neonates.
- The stomach herniates through the oesophageal hiatus, which can be rolling or sliding.

A/R: Previous affected sibling, CHD (25%), renal anomalies, persistent pulmonary hypertension of the newborn.
DD: pneumothorax, congenital cystic adenomatoid malformation.

E: 1/2000–4000 live births. M : F = 1.5 : 1. Accounts for 8% of all major congenital anomalies.

H&E: May have a history of polyhydramnios, and most commonly present with a history of cyanosis and respiratory distress in the immediate neonatal period. If there is a left-sided posterolateral hernia, there may be poor air entry on the left and a shift of cardiac sounds into the right chest.

P: See **A**.

I: **Antenatal USS:** usually diagnosed on routine antenatal scans.
Karyotype: chromosomal studies.
Radiology: CXR (with prior placing of an NG tube to aid gastric positioning), cardiac echo, renal USS.

M: **Medical:**

- Intubation and mechanical ventilation are required for all infants with severe CDH (bag and mask positive-pressure ventilation should be avoided).
- Insert NG tube to decompress bowel, central venous catheter and arterial line for intensive monitoring.
- The lungs are immature and may be surfactant deficient; administration of exogenous surfactant can be used.

Surgical:

- After resuscitation and stabilisation of the neonate, the diaphragmatic defect is closed with or without the need for a synthetic patch.

Post-operatively: High-frequency oscillation, NO and ECMO may be of benefit.

C: Pulmonary hypoplasia, intestinal malrotation (30–60%), gastric and midgut volvulus, gastric or other GI perforations, bilateral renal hypertrophy.

P: Reported mortality is 50–60%.

Hernias, inguinal and umbilical

D: Protrusion of bowel through a defect in the anterior abdominal wall.

A: **Inguinal hernias:**

- Usually indirect in children.
- The processus vaginalis is an outpouching of peritoneum that is attached to the testicle and trails behind it as it descends retroperitoneally into the scrotum *in utero*. When the processus vaginalis does not obliterate during gestation, a congenital inguinal hernia results.

Umbilical hernias:

- During gestation the abdominal organs are formed outside of the foetus's body and return to the abdominal cavity around the 10th week.
- If the muscles of the abdominal wall fail to close around the abdominal organs, an umbilical hernia may form.

A/R: Preterm infants, low birth weight, family history of childhood hernias, Ehlers–Danlos syndrome, CF, connective tissue disorders, and conditions that ↑ intra-abdominal pressure.

E: **Inguinal hernias:** 1–5% of children. M > F. **Peak age:** < 2 years. R > L. 10% of children develop hernia on the opposite side, 20% of preterm infants.
Umbilical hernias: 15% of children, M = F. **Peak age:** at birth or in 1st few weeks. African-American > Caucasian children.

H&E: **Inguinal hernia:** examine patient in supine and standing position. Feel for a swelling in the groin that has an expansible cough impulse and does not transilluminate. Indirect hernias may extend into the scrotum. They are reducible by manipulation unless incarcerated (tender, firm mass), when signs and symptoms of intestinal obstruction may occur (rare in umbilical hernias).
Umbilical hernia: appears as a bulge at the umbilicus.
DD of inguinal hernia: hydrocoele, retractile testes, undescended testes, femoral hernias, and lymph nodes.

P: See **A**.

I: Diagnosis is usually clinical.
USS: only if diagnosis is in doubt, (difficulty distinguishing between a hernia and a hydrocoele).

M: **Inguinal hernia:** elective surgery is performed as a day case under general anaesthesia; protruding bowel is reduced into the abdominal cavity and the processus vaginalis is closed. Consider bilateral repair due to the common occurrence of bilateral hernias.
Umbilical hernia: most umbilical hernias do not need to be repaired. The opening in the abdominal muscles will usually close over a few months to years. However, if the defect is > 1.5 cm in diameter, or the child is > 5 years it is unlikely to spontaneously heal and will need to be surgically repaired.

C: **Inguinal hernias:** 15–60% of infants < 1 year with hernias will develop incarceration, requiring emergency reduction and repair. The prevention of these emergency operations is the goal of elective hernia repair at the earliest convenience of the family.
Umbilical hernias: risk of incarceration is very low.

P: Excellent following surgery. Higher risk of surgical complications in incarcerated hernias.

D: Infection by HSV1 or HSV2.

A: **Routes of transmission:**
Neonatal HSV: due to infant exposure to shedding of HSV2 in the maternal cervical canal during vaginal delivery.
Childhood HSV: transmitted through intimate contact (e.g. saliva) with an affected individual who is actively shedding the virus; usually HSV1.
Genital HSV: HSV2 (75%), HSV1 (25%). May occur in adolescents due to ↑sexual activity.

A/R: **Neonatal HSV:** 1° maternal infection, PROM.
Childhood HSV: crowded living environment.
Genital HSV: early sexual contacts, promiscuity.

E: **Neonatal HSV:** 1–2/5000 live births.
Childhood HSV: 20–30% of children exhibit HSV1 by 5 years of age.
Genital HSV: 25% of adolescent and adults.

H&E: **Neonatal HSV:** vesicles on skin/mucous membranes appear in only 30%; therefore diagnosis may not be apparent. Presentation ranges from lethargy, poor feeding, and irritability to encephalitis with seizures, pneumonitis, and disseminated multiorgan involvement.
Childhood HSV: usually asymptomatic but may present with;

- **Gingivostomatitis:** usually occurs at 10 months to 3 years with painful vesicles on lips, gums, and anterior surface of tongue and hard palate, odynophagia, and a high fever.
- **Ocular manifestation:** conjunctivitis, keratoconjunctivitis (inflammation of the cornea and conjunctiva) and dendritic ulcers of the cornea.
- **Eczema herpeticum:** large numbers of vesicular lesions on eczematous skin; may result in electrolyte imbalances and 2° bacterial infection.
- **Herpetic whitlow:** painful erythematous, oedematous white pustules at the site of broken skin on hands and fingers.
- **Common 'cold sore':** painful vesicles on the vermillion (mucocutaneous) border of lips 2° to reactivation of the virus.

Genital HSV: erythematous vesicles, which ulcerate on the penis, perineum, and anus in males, and on the cervix and external genitalia in females.

P: HSV is a double-stranded DNA virus. Virus enters via mucous membranes or skin. Once infected, majority carry the virus in a latent form within the dorsal root ganglia.

I: **Microscopy:** vesicular scrapings show multinuclear giant cells and intranuclear inclusions.
ELISA/immunofluorescence: HSV1 and 2 antibodies in the blood.
PCR: tests for HSV1 and HSV2 DNA from CSF, conjunctiva, stool, urine, and anogenital mucosa.
Slit lamp examination: to exclude dendritic ulcers in ocular HSV.

M: **IV acyclovir:** in neonatal HSV, disseminated disease, or encephalitis.
Topical acyclovir: cold sores and stomatitis.

C: Encephalitis, viral meningitis (usually HSV2), bacterial superinfection in genital HSV. Corneal ulceration can → scarring and loss of vision.

P: **Neonatal HSV:** 80% mortality if left untreated, still 50% if treated.
Childhood and adolescent HSV: usually self-limiting, lasting 1–2 weeks but may re-occur in a third of cases.

Hirschsprung disease

D: Congenital condition which results in obstruction of the large intestine 2° to abnormal intestinal motility.
Short-segment disease (75%): affects only the rectum and sigmoid.
Long-segment disease (10%): affects the entire colon.

A: During normal development neural crest-derived ganglion cells migrate from proximal to distal bowel. In Hirschsprung disease the cells do not complete their migration, leaving the rectum and sometimes the colon without parasympathetic nerve innervation. The affected bowel therefore has only sympathetic nerve innervation, which → hypertonicity and lack of appropriate relaxation in response to proximal distension. This results in a narrow and contracted segment of bowel and stasis of stool in the bowel proximal to this.

A/R: Down, Waardenburg syndrome, ↑familial incidence in long-segment disease.

E: 1/5000 live births; accounts for 20% of all neonatal obstruction. **Sex:** M : F = 3 : 1. **Age of presentation:** < 1 month (80%), < 1 year (95%).

H: **Neonatal presentation:**
(1) Failure to pass meconium in < 24 h.
(2) Acute intestinal obstruction; abdominal distension, poor feeding, bilious vomiting.
(3) Severe life-threatening enterocolitis 2° to *Clostridium difficile* infection.
Infantile presentation:
(1) Chronic constipation with abdominal distension without soiling.
(2) Intermittent abdominal pain and fever during episodes of retained faeces.
(3) Failure to thrive.

E: Palpable stools throughout or in the left lower abdomen. Rectal examination reveals an empty rectum with normal anal tone. A narrowed segment of bowel may be felt. Following rectal examination an explosive gush of stool and flatus may occur.

P: Rectal mucosa and submucosa demonstrate the absence of ganglion cells with ↑amounts of acetylcholinesterase-stained nerve endings.

I: **AXR:** dilated bowel loops and fluid levels.
Anorectal manometry: pressure at the internal and external anal sphincters is measured in response to transient rectal distension. With rectal distension there is usually a reflex relaxation of the internal sphincter and contraction of the external sphincter. In Hirschsprung's disease the internal sphincter does not relax but remains contracted. A negative result rules out Hirschsprung's disease. A positive result is an indication for a rectal biopsy.
Barium study: to estimate the length of the aganglionic segment.

M: **Surgery:**
1st stage: colostomy just above the transition to allow decompression of the proximally dilated colon.
2nd stage (at 3–6 months): rectosigmoidectomy and anastomosis of normally innervated bowel to anus. The colostomy is then closed.
Short-segment disease: may be treated with anal dilatation and upper partial sphincterotomy.

C: NEC, post-op complications including anal stenosis, faecal incontinence, stricture, prolapse, and perianal abscesses.

P: Good in the absence of enterocolitis. There are often ongoing problems with defaecation and incontinence in spite of/after surgery.

Human immunodeficiency virus (HIV)

D: Virus that infects and disables the host's CD4 T cells.

A: **Vertical transmission (most common cause):** *in utero*, perinatally or via breastfeeding.
Sexual transmission: abuse in children, intercourse in adolescents.
IV drug abuse: rare in children.

A/R: Risk of vertical transmission is higher with high maternal HIV titres and advanced disease.

E: 2 000 000 children worldwide are suspected to be infected with HIV.
Higher rates of prevalence within children from ethnic minority groups.

H&E: **Asymptomatic or non-specific:** lymphadenopathy, parotitis, hepatosplenomegaly, recurrent bacterial infections.
Candidiasis: oral; white/yellow plaques or well-circumscribed erythematous areas and loss of tongue papillae. Oesophageal; dysphagia, odynophagia, and retrosternal pain.
Herpes simplex: herpes labialis, gingivostomatitis, oesophagitis, or chronic erosive vesicles on the skin.
VZV: recurrent/persistent vesicular eruptions. Severe infection with scarring, hyperkeratotic, haemorrhagic lesions involving >1 dermatome.
Human papillomavirus: flat warts covering large areas of the forehead, the temples, the neck, and the upper body.
Neoplasms: NHL, Burkitt's lymphoma, Kaposi's sarcoma.
AIDS: PCP, severe failure to thrive, encephalopathy.

P: Virus enters CD4 lymphocytes by binding with CD4 and a chemokine receptor using its glycoprotein receptor (gp120). Viral reverse transcriptase converts RNA to DNA, which is incorporated into the host genome.

I: **Serology:** HIV antibodies at >18 months when maternal antibodies have disappeared. **PCR:** to detect HIV DNA prior to this age.
Assess severity: viral load/HIV RNA, and CD4 count.
Endoscopy: if oesophageal candidiasis is suspected.
Screen for other diseases: TB (Mantoux's test), hepatitis B/C (serology), syphilis, and toxoplasmosis.

M: **Prevention:**
(1) Mothers with HIV should not breastfeed their child (UK guidelines). 25–40% transmission amongst breastfed children, ↓ to ~15% when breastfeeding is avoided.
(2) Reduce maternal viral load with antiretroviral drugs antenatally, perinatally, and postnatally; reduces transmission rate to 5%.
(3) Elective Caesarean section to avoid contact with the birth canal; reduces transmission rate to 1% (less with low maternal viral load).

Prophylaxis: co-trimoxazole against PCP, give all immunisations except BCG, which can disseminate, and pneumococcal vaccine.
Screen for opportunistic infection regularly.
Regular monitoring: viral load/CD4 count. Start antiretroviral therapy if these indicators of disease progression start to deteriorate:
(1) Nucleoside analogue reverse transcriptase inhibitors (zidovudine).
(2) Non-nucleoside reverse transcriptase inhibitors (nevirapine).
(3) Protease inhibitors (indinavir).

C: Drug side-effects, e.g. myelosuppression with zidovudine. Opportunistic infections with progression of disease.

P: Viral load/plasma HIV RNA, and CD4 counts correlate well with disease progression and long-term prognosis.

Hydrocephalus

D: Excess CSF from abnormal flow, absorption, or production.

A: **Obstructive hydrocephalus:** disruption in the flow of CSF within the ventricular system.

(1) **Aqueductal stenosis or atresia:** commonest site of intraventricular obstruction in infants with congenital hydrocephalus.
(2) **Obstruction of the 4th ventricle:** Dandy–Walker syndrome (cystic dilatation of the 4th ventricle with cerebellar hypoplasia).
(3) **Obstruction due to intracranial mass lesion:** tumours of the posterior fossa (medulloblastoma, astrocytomas, ependymoma), haematomas, galanic vein aneurysm.

Communicating hydrocephalus: disruption in the flow of CSF in the surface pathways.

(1) **Arnold–Chiari malformations:** herniation of cerebellar tonsils through the foramen magnum; frequently associated with neural tube defects:
   - Myelomeningocele: outpouching of the spinal cord through the posterior bony vertebral column.
   - Cranial meningocele: meningeal sac protrudes through a skull defect.
(2) **Encephalocele:** protrusion of cerebral tissue through midline cranial defect located in frontal or occipital regions.
(3) **Meningeal adhesions:** 2° to inflammation (meningitis) or haemorrhage (intraventricular or subarachnoid).

↑Production of CSF:
Choroid plexus papilloma: rare cause of hydrocephalus.

A/R: Family history, NF.

E: **Congenital hydrocephalus:** 3–5/1000 live births.

H: **Infants:**
Slow progression: infants may thrive and develop normally apart from poor head control.
Rapid progression: irritability, lethargy, failure to gain weight, vomiting.
Older children:
Posterior fossa tumours: cerebellar signs; ataxic gait, dyspraxia, slurred speech.
'Arrested' hydrocephalus: 'cocktail party' syndrome; talkative and jovial child but lacking in concentration and depth.

E: **Signs of hydrocephalus include:**

(1) Progressive ↑ in occipitofrontal head circumference or $>$ 97th centile.
(2) Wide open bulging anterior fontanelle.
(3) Widening of the coronal, sagittal, and lambdoidal sutures.
(4) Eyes deviate downwards ('setting-sun' sign).
(5) Papilloedema is uncommon in congenital hydrocephalus.

P: Accumulation of CSF in a confined space → ↑intraventricular pressure and raised ICP. In infants there is initial compensation from open fontanelles.

I: **CT/USS:** may show dilatation of ventricles and any tumours or cysts present.
MRI: shows greater anatomical detail, and with contrast illustrates flow through the aqueduct.

M: **Surgical:** insertion of a shunt with a one-way valve from the ventricle to the peritoneum (or the right atrium).
Supportive: requires long-term multidisciplinary follow-up to provide support for neurological sequelae.

C: **Shunt complications:** obstruction, infection, especially *Staphylococcus epidermidis*, and overdrainage, which can → subdural haemorrhages.
Long-term sequelae: global developmental delay, impaired memory and vision, precocious puberty.

P: Some forms of hydrocephalus are temporary, such as meningeal adhesion 2° to infection or haemorrhage; some forms give rise to limited ventricular enlargement and then cease; compensated hydrocephalus. However, in most cases the ventricles will continue to enlarge and compress brain matter, resulting in a very poor prognosis.

Hyperthyroidism

D: Overactivity of the thyroid gland, which → an increase in levels of circulating T_3 and T_4.

A: **1° Graves' disease:** autoimmune hyperthyroidism due to the production of TSIs that stimulate the thyroid gland.
Transient neonatal hyperthyroidism: 2° to maternal Graves' disease; circulating TSIs cross the placenta and stimulate the foetal thyroid.
Permanent neonatal hyperthyroidism: germline mutation in the TSH receptor results in its constitutive activation. Autosomal dominant or *de novo* mutation.

A/R: Excessive growth or tall stature.

E: **1° Graves' disease:** peak in teenage years, very rare in early childhood. M : F = 1 : 5.
Transient neonatal hyperthyroidism: incidence 1/50 000 live births; 1–2% of neonates of mothers with Graves' disease will be affected.
Permanent neonatal hyperthyroidism: rare.

H: Anxiety, restlessness, weight loss, rapid growth in height, advanced bone maturity, learning difficulties/behavioural problems, psychosis.

E: **1° Graves' disease:** the clinical features in children are similar to those of adults although the eye signs are less common.
General: sweating, diarrhoea, weight loss, tremor, tachycardia with a wide pulse pressure, warm vasodilated peripheries, goitre.
Eye signs: exophthalmos, ophthalmoplegia, lid retraction, lid lag.
Transient neonatal hyperthyroidism: irritability, weight loss, diarrhoea, and exophthalmos.

P: **Graves' disease:** TSIs act on the TSH-receptor as an autoimmune phenomenon due to interactions between T and B lymphocytes. Eye symptoms are caused by mucopolysaccharides and lymphocytes infiltrating the orbital, skin, and SC tissues.

I: **Antenatal monitoring:** CTG trace will indicate tachycardia in foetuses of affected mothers.
Graves' disease: $\uparrow T_4 +/- \uparrow T_3$, TSH levels are highly suppressed ($< 0.1 \mu U/L$), and antithyroid peroxisomal antibodies may be present.
Transient neonatal hyperthyroidism: presence of TSIs in the blood, $\uparrow T_4$, and $\uparrow T_3$.

M: **Medical treatment:**
(1) Carbimazole or propylthiouracil are the 1st line treatment options.
(2) β-blockers are given for symptomatic relief of tremor, anxiety, and tachycardia, and to protect the patient from cardiac arrhythmias.
Treatment usually lasts for 2 years. 40–75% of patients relapse when medical treatment is stopped; these patients either need a 2nd course of medical therapy, radioiodine treatment or surgery.
Radioiodine treatment: highly successful although it may cause hypothyroidism and require subsequent lifelong treatment with T_4.
Surgical: subtotal thyroidectomy is indicated if there is failure of medical management and in permanent neonatal hyperthyroidism as 1st line treatment.

C: **Cardiac arrhythmias:** important and life-threatening complication.
Complications of treatment: some patients will become hypothyroid with treatment and will therefore require T_4 replacement therapy for life.

P: In all cases prompt treatment is of paramount importance to prevent complications. Following successful treatment there is good prognosis with a normal life expectancy.

Hypoglycaemia in neonates

D: Abnormally low glucose levels can cause an encephalopathy and have the potential to produce long-term neurological injury. It is difficult to establish the exact level at which this neurological injury occurs. Definition of hypoglycaemia is <2.6 mmol/L.

A: Neonatal hypoglycaemia can either be transient or persistent, and can be subdivided into ketotic or non-ketotic causes.
Ketotic cause: usually due to ↓ production/supply of glucose.
Non-ketotic cause: due to an ↑ in insulin production.
Transient ketotic hypoglycaemia: 'at-risk' groups: IUGR, preterm infants, intrauterine or perinatal trauma, cerebral hypoxia or malformation, and sepsis.
Transient non-ketotic hypoglycaemia: infants with diabetic mothers, severe Rh disease, Beckwith–Wiedemann syndrome (exomphalos, macroglossia, and gigantism).
Persistent ketotic hypoglycaemia: enzyme defects either direct (GSDs) or indirect (galactosaemia/fructose intolerance), hormone deficiency (GH/glucocorticoids).
Persistent non-ketotic hypoglycaemia: islet cell hyperplasia with or without Beckwith–Wiedemann syndrome, discrete adenoma, nesidioblastosis (↑islet cells throughout the pancreas).

A/R: Neonatal seizures.

E: Now much less common due to ↑ vigilance in the postnatal period.

H&E: **General:** irritability, apnoea, lethargy, hypothermia, seizures.
Specific: macrosomia (hyperinsulinism), jaundice (in galactosaemia or sepsis), hepatomegaly (GSDs).

P: **Preterm and growth-restricted neonates:** due to ↓glycogen stores and impaired ability to produce a ketone (an alternative brain fuel) in response to low glucose levels.
Neonates with diabetic mothers: due to hyperplasia of the islet cells in the pancreas, which causes high insulin levels (due to high circulating glucose levels in utero).

I: **Routine bloods:** ↓glucose, ↑ketones (in ketotic hypoglycaemia), FBC, CRP.
Specific bloods: insulin (hyperinsulinism), cortisol (hypoadrenalism), GH (hypopituitarism), lactate (Type I and V GSDs).
Urine analysis: for ketones.

M: **Mildly symptomatic infants:** if no contraindications to feeding, hypoglycaemia is managed with ↑enteral feeds. At-risk infants should be monitored until their blood sugar stabilises.
Severely symptomatic infants, refractory hypoglycaemia, or contra-indications to feeding:
(1) IV dextrose; a bolus of 2–5 ml/kg of 10% dextrose may be required followed by an infusion to prevent rebound hypoglycaemia.
(2) If increase in glucose intake is required, the volume of the fluid should be increased rather than its concentration wherever possible to avoid cerebral oedema.
(3) If the baby requires > 10 mg/kg/min IV dextrose infusion, consider:
- Glucagon IM if no venous access or IV.
- Diazoxide and chlorothiazide in suspected hyperinsulinism.
- Hydrocortisone if adrenal insufficiency is suspected.

Surgery: may be required for nesidioblastosis/islet cell adenoma.

C: Prolonged symptomatic hypoglycaemia can cause permanent neurological disability.

P: The prognosis is good with prompt recognition and treatment.

Hypospadias

D: A congenital malformation of the urethral groove and urethral canal, resulting in an abnormal opening on the ventral penile surface. Associated abnormal curvature of the penis or 'chordee' is common.
Classification:
(1) According to position of the urethral meatus.
(2) Glandular, coronal, subcoronal, midpenile, scrotal, and perineal.
(3) 60% are distal, 25% are subcoronal or midpenile, 15% are proximal.

A: There is incomplete development of the prepuce, termed dorsal hood, in which the foreskin is on the dorsal aspect of the penile shaft and absent ventrally.

A/R: Although it is usually an isolated anomaly, hypospadias is common in boys with multiple congenital anomalies; 10% have cryptorchidism, and inguinal hernias are also common.

E: Hypospadias is the most common anomaly of the urethra in males; 1/250 live births.

H&E: Found at birth. Boys with hypospadias will have difficulty in directing their urinary stream. Depending on the severity of the anomaly, it may be necessary to void in a sitting position. Constriction of the abnormal opening → partial urinary obstruction and is associated with an ↑incidence of UTIs.

P: See **A**.

I: **Karyotype:** in midpenile hypospadias and cryptorchidism.
Imaging: patients with penoscrotal hypospadias should undergo a micturating cytourethrogram.

M: **Treatment:** surgical urethroplasty to construct a new distal urethra and repair abnormal curvature of the penis. Surgery can be performed at 6–12 months and preferably before 3 years of age.
Type of repair: depends on the severity of the defect.
(1) Mild defects may be repaired in a single operation as an outpatient.
(2) Severe defects may require 2 or more procedures.
Parents should be strongly advised to avoid circumcision prior to surgery as the foreskin may be used in reconstruction; a small piece of foreskin is used to create a tube to extend the urethral length and allow placement of the urethral opening at the tip of the penis.
Follow-up: with appropriate imaging to exclude complications of surgical procedure.

C: **If left untreated:**
(1) Deformity of urinary stream.
(2) Sexual dysfunction 2° to penile dysfunction.
(3) Subfertility if the urethral meatus is proximal (near penile base) as normal ejaculation and insemination is partially or totally prevented.
(4) Meatal stenosis.
Complication rate for surgery:
(1) $<5\%$ for distal hypospadias.
(2) 5–10% for midpenile hypospadias.
(3) 15% for proximal hypospadias.
Surgical complications: urethrocutaneous fistula, haematoma, wound infection, meatal stenosis.

P: Good with appropriate surgical reconstruction and follow-up.
Distal hypospadias has a better outcome than proximal.

Hypoxic–ischaemic encephalopathy (HIE)

D: Clinical manifestation of brain injury immediately or up to 48 h after asphyxia, whether antenatal, intrapartum, or postnatal.

A: Occurs following perinatal events that reduce oxygen and glucose delivery to the brain. These factors are often interrelated. The exact pathology is unclear but involves excitatory neurotransmitters (glutamate, glycine), cell death by apoptosis, and an inflammatory reaction.

A/R: **Obstructive labour:** malpresentation, cephalopelvic disproportion, multiple births (particularly in the 2nd twin due to prolapsed cord or malpresentation), postmature neonates.
Hypotension: maternal haemorrhage (placental abruption, placenta praevia).
Hypertension: fulminant pregnancy-induced hypertension and related seizures.
Infants at risk: preterm infants, congenital cardiac disorders.

E: 2–4/1000 live births.

H: Determine risk factors and difficulties during neonatal resuscitation; persistently low APGAR scores, delayed respiratory effort, ventilatory disturbances (i.e. apnea, respiratory failure), depressed level of consciousness, and seizures.

E: **Classification of HIE:**
Stage 1: hyperalert (eyes wide open, ↓blinking, excessive response to stimulation), impaired feeding 2° to weak suck but normal tone.
Stage 2: lethargic, mild hypotonia, reduced spontaneous movement, seizures.
Stage 3: no spontaneous movements, withdrawal or decerebrate posturing only to pain, variable abnormal tone (hypotonia/hypertonia), suppression of primitive (Moro's, tonic neck, sucking) and brainstem (corneal, gag) reflexes. Prolonged seizures refractory to treatment +/− multiorgan failure.

P: See **A**.

I: **CTG:** there is poor correlation between specific patterns and neurological outcome.
Foetal cord pH: poor association of low pH and long-term neurological outcome. Most neurologically symptomatic neonates are not markedly acidotic and most acidotic newborns are not neurologically symptomatic.
EEG: becomes progressively more abnormal with worsening HIE although it does return to normal over the subsequent days/weeks.
CT/MRI brain: detects focal, multifocal, and generalised ischaemic lesions, and may also detect IVH.
LP: to exclude meningitis/haemorrhage.

M: **Prevention:** good antenatal care, detection and management of maternal medical conditions, prompt recognition and appropriate intervention for significant foetal distress.
Neonatal resuscitation: (see chapter).
Prevention of 2° CNS insults: seizure control with anticonvulsants, correction of hypoglycemia, hypotension, hyponatraemia (slowly), hypocalcaemia, and hypomagnesaemia, control of brain oedema, prevention of fluid overload, appropriate oxygenation +/− ventilation.
Developmental follow-up: close monitoring in consultation with a developmental specialist or neurologist. Patients with motor, speech, or learning disabilities need serial testing and input from occupational, physical, and speech therapists.

C: HIE may result even if managed aggressively as most asphyxia occurs before and not after birth.

The combination of EEG and neurological examination has been shown to give the best correlation with outcome.

Stage 1: 90% have a good outcome.

Stage 2: 40–50% have normal neurological outcome.

Stage 3: 90% have major neurological sequelae; microcephaly, global developmental delay, cerebral palsy, and epilepsy.

D: **SIgAD:** virtual absence of serum and secretory IgA.
SCID: deficiency and defects in T-cell and B-cell function, which → impaired cell-mediated and Ig-mediated immunity.
XLA: lack of mature B cells; there is virtually no serum Ig, but cell-mediated immune function is normal. T-cell numbers and function are normal.
Syndromes:
(1) Wiskott–Aldrich syndrome: T-cell dysfunction, thrombocytopaenia.
(2) Di George syndrome: absent thymus and parathyroids, midline facial clefts, CHD.

A: **SIgAD:** autosomal dominant condition or acquired after viral infections.
SCID: 50% X-linked recessive, 50% autosomal recessive gene mutations.
XLA: mutation in the X-linked tyrosine kinase gene expressed in early B lymphocytes.

A/R: **SIgAD + XLA:** autoimmune disease (SLE, rheumatoid-like arthritis).
XLA: inflammatory bowel disease.

E: **SIgAD:** 1–2/1000, commonest inherited immunodeficiency.
SCID: 1–2/75 000, most severe of all immunodeficiencies.
XLA: 1/90 000, only in males.

H&E: **SIgAD:** usually asymptomatic; however, may have recurrent sinopulmonary and GI infections and are prone to respiratory tract allergies.
SCID: recurrent bacterial, viral, and fungal infections in early infancy.
XLA: recurrent bacterial infections begin after 6 months of age due to ↓maternal antibodies.

P: **SIgAD:** failure of maturation of IgA B cells. Immature forms are present in normal numbers.
SCID: absent or immature lymph nodes, tonsils, adenoids, and Peyer's patches. Patients have very small but histologically normal thymuses, and the spleen is depleted of lymphocytes.
XLA: pre-B lymphocytes are present in normal numbers in the marrow, but lymph nodes and the spleen lack germinal centres, and plasma cells are absent from all tissues.

I: **Bloods:** ↓WCC (SCID), ↑ESR (autoimmune disease, chronic infection).
Serology:
- **SIgAD:** IgA < 5 mg/L.
- **SCID:** low/absent Igs, no antibodies following immunisation.
- **XLA:** IgG < 100 mg/dl after 6 months with absent IgM and IgA.

CXR: absent thymus (SCID), signs of infection.
Exclude other disorders: Howell–Jolly bodies in asplenia.

M: **SIgAD:** antibiotics for recurrent bacterial URTIs, e.g. sinusitis.
SCID: only treatment option is BMT or gene therapy.
XLA: IV Ig every 3–4 weeks forms the mainstay of treatment; supplementary antibiotics, bronchodilators, and steroid inhalers in children with CLD.

C: **SCID:** opportunistic infections (candida, EBV) can be fatal.
XLA: bronchiectasis, malnutrition from inflammatory bowel disease, meningoencephalitis from enteroviral infection, ↑incidence of lymphoma.

P: **SIgAD:** good, except when patients have associated autoimmune disease (SLE, rheumatoid-like arthritis).
SCID: 95% success if HLA-matched BMT is performed at < 3 months.
XLA: recurrent bacteria pneumonias are the leading cause of mortality. Patients who receive Ig before the age of 5 years have the best outcome.

Impetigo

D: Contagious superficial infection of the skin. There are 2 forms:
Bullous impetigo (30% of cases): blistering form.
Nonbullous impetigo (70% of cases): crusted form.

A: **Bullous:** results from invasion by phage group II strains of *Staphylococcus aureus* onto either intact or disrupted skin. This occurs after colonisation of the URT, usually involving the nasopharyngeal tract.
Nonbullous: in both developing and developed countries, group A β-haemolytic streptococcus is the primary pathogen. However, in developed countries *Staph. aureus* is responsible in up to 50% of cases. Bacteria invade disrupted skin 2° to eczema, insect bites, abrasions, varicella lesions, or other trauma.

A/R: High temperature or humidity, recent antibiotic treatment, immunocompromise.

E: Commonest skin infection in children today.
Bullous: affects neonates and older children.
Nonbullous: affects 2–5-year-old children.

H&E: **Bullous:** usually has a history of disseminated 1–2 cm thin-roofed bullae that rupture spontaneously without a history of localised lymphadenopathy or cutaneous disruption. Lesions are most commonly found on the face.
Nonbullous: a tiny pustule or honey-coloured crusted plaque forms following a break in the skin and spreads rapidly with occasional associated pruritis. Regional lymphadenopathy occurs in 90% of cases. Lesions may be found on the face, trunk, extremities, buttocks, and perineum.

P: **Bullous:** an epidermolytic toxin is thought to disrupt epidermal cell attachments and allow *S. aureus* to invade intact skin.
Nonbullous: organisms directly penetrate epidermis superficially. Dermal vessels dilate and upper dermis fills with migrating polymorphs. Collections of pus form in the stratum corneum; these pustules rupture rapidly.

I: Diagnosis is based mainly on history and examination of lesions.
Bacterial culture: exudates of nose to determine whether patient is *S. aureus* carrier.

M: **Local wound care:** application of wet dressings to affected areas to aid removal of the honey-coloured crusts in nonbullous impetigo.
Topical antibiotic treatment: topical mupirocin is considered the treatment of choice for individuals with uncomplicated localised impetigo.
Systemic antibiotic treatment: oral flucloxacillin +/− penicillin V (if nonbullous) should be used in infections that are widespread, complicated, or have systemic manifestations.
Prevention of spread:

- School/nursery exclusion until lesions are healed/treated and dry.
- Nasal carriage of *S. aureus* (15–20%) can be eradicated with nasal cream containing mupirocin.

C: Acute post-streptococcal GN is a rare but serious complication of nonbullous impetigo 2° to group A β-haemolytic streptococcus infection. It occurs ~3 weeks after onset of skin lesions and is due to antibody response to a kidney antigen that crossreacts with a streptococcal antigen.

P: Good with appropriate treatment.

D: Ingestion of harmful substances by children unaware of the consequences.

A: **Wide variety:** iron tablets, alcohol, paracetamol, acids, alkalis, salicylates, OCPs, sleeping tablets, antidepressants. Between 2 and 4 years, chemicals such as lavatory cleaners and polish are likely causes.

A/R: Environmental factors, poor supervision of children.

E: **Peak age:** $2\frac{1}{2}$ years – age of the inquisitive toddler.

H: **Elicit a thorough history:** exact time of ingestion, estimated amount and method of ingestion. Assess whether there are any inconsistencies in the history; warning signs of abuse. Check if child is on the Child Protection Register. Determine any medical conditions affecting the child.

E: **Depends on substance ingested:** vomiting, unusual sleepiness, diarrhoea, breathing difficulties, bleeding, confusion, coma, convulsions, hypotension, tachycardia, arrhythmias. Chemical burns around mouth and lips.

P: Dependent on individual poison.

I: **Iron:** AXR, serum levels of iron and glucose.
Alcohol: blood glucose, alcohol.
Paracetamol: plasma concentration 4 h post ingestion, LFTs, INR.
Acids/alkalis: early upper GI endoscopy.
Salicylates: glucose, U&Es, LFTs, INR, ABG, salicylate level (repeat after 2 h due to continued absorption).

M: **Resuscitate:** ABC.
Assess toxicity of poison: contact any Poison Centre in the UK, e.g. Guy's Hospital for specialist advice or access the website TOXBASE.
Gastric decontamination: lavage, activated charcoal; usually performed within 1 h of ingestion. If unconscious, there is significant risk of aspiration pneumonia. Avoid in acid/alkali ingestion.
Prevention: all inadvertant poisoning should be followed up by health visitor.
(1) Child-resistant packaging; however, do not rely on child-proof containers.
(2) Take medications away from bedside or bags; locked cabinet is ideal.
(3) Throw away old or unwanted drugs or return to pharmacist.
(4) Ensure supervision if child is in kitchen or bathroom.
Specific measures:
(1) Iron: desferrioxamine antidote.
(2) Paracetamol: N-acetylcysteine.
(3) Salicylates: alkaline diuresis +/− renal dialysis may be required in severe cases.
(4) Acid/alkali ingestion: steroids may reduce inflammation.
General measures: observation with monitoring of vital function may be all that is required.

C: **Iron:** metabolic acidosis, liver failure, hypoglycaemia, gastric strictures, and multiorgan failure.
Alcohol: hypoglycaemia and respiratory failure.
Paracetamol: gastric irritation, liver failure, multiorgan failure.
Acids/alkalis: ulceration and then stenosis of upper GI tract.
Salicylates: hearing impairment, hypoglycaemia, respiratory alkalosis followed by metabolic acidosis, cardiac depression, pulmonary oedema and/or hepatic encephalopathy (Reye's syndrome).

P: Recovery is expected in most cases if vital functions are not affected.

Inborn errors of amino acid metabolism

D: Hereditary biochemical disorders resulting from a mutation in a gene important in amino acid metabolism.

A:

PKU	**Autosomal recessive mutation → either:** (1) **Classical:** complete or near-complete deficiency of phenylalanine hydroxylase, required for the degradation of phenylalanine down the tyrosine pathway; **or** (2) **Hyperphenylalaninemia:** due to deficiency of the phenylalanine hydroxylase cofactor.
Homocystinuria	3 types; most commonly due to cystathionine synthase deficiency; homocystinuria type 1.
OCA	**2 genetically distinct autosomal recessive forms:** **OCAI:** gene defect on the long arm of chromosome 11, encoding the enzyme tyrosinase. **OCAII:** most common form of generalised albinism due to a gene defect on chromosome 15 → absence in the protein required for transport of tyrosine across the melanosome membrane.

A/R: Chromosomal abnormalities, e.g. Prader–Willi and Angelman syndrome that have deletions on chromosome 15 may also have OCAII.

E: **PKU:** 1/15 000 live births. **Homocystinuria:** 1/344 000 live births. **OCAI:** 1/40 000 live births. **OCAII:** 1/15 000 live births.

H:

PKU	**Infants:** normal at birth, gradual development of cognitive impairment if untreated, lose 4 IQ points/month, severe vomiting. **Older children:** hyperactive, purposeless movements, rhythmic rocking and athetosis, severe learning disability.
Homocystinuria	Normal at birth. **Infants:** nonspecific; failure to thrive, developmental delay, and convulsions. **>3 years old:** subluxation of ocular lens → severe myopia. Later, astigmatism, glaucoma, retinal detachment, and optic atrophy. Progressive cognitive impairment and thromboembolic episodes are common.
OCA	Lack of pigment evident at birth; photophobia, ↓visual acuity, absent binocular vision. Blindness and skin cancer are major late sequelae in severe forms. OCAII is milder than OCAI.

E:

PKU	Blonder than siblings, fair skin, and blue eyes, may have seborrhoeic/eczematoid skin rash, unpleasant odour of phenylacetic acid (musty), hypertonic with hyperactive deep tendon reflexes. NB: clinical manifestations are rarely seen in countries where neonatal screening programmes exist.

Homocystinuria Skeletal abnormalities: tall and thin with elongated limbs and arachnodactyly, high-arched palate, genu valgum and pes cavus.

OCA Lack of skin, eye, and hair pigmentation, strabismus, presence of red reflex, pink translucent iris at birth that may change to blue or brown with age.

I:

Classical PKU **Guthrie test:** elevated levels of phenylalanine after 48–72 h of life, raised plasma phenylalanine, ↑urinary levels of phenylalanine metabolites, normal tyrosine and cofactor levels.

Homocystinuria Elevation of methionine and homocysteine in plasma and urine. Generalised osteoporosis is the main radiographic finding.

OCA Genetic analysis.

M:

PKU Lifelong phenylalanine-free diet to maintain blood levels below 0.6–0.8 mmol/L. Levels should be monitored 2 – 3×/week at onset, then 1×/week after 1 year.

Homocystinuria Pyridoxine (100–500 mg/day) and folic acid (10–20 mg/day). All animal proteins should be withheld; plant sources are acceptable. Betaine is used to recycle homocysteine to methionine. Dipyridamole or low-dose aspirin for anticoagulation. OCP should be avoided.

OCA Avoid sunlight, sun protection, tinted glasses, regular ophthalmic and dermatological review.

C:

PKU Reduced IQ. If diagnosis and treatment are delayed, permanent brain damage is likely to occur. There is CNS deterioration if the special diet is stopped.

Homocystinuria Recently raised homocysteine has been recognised as a risk factor for IHD and thromboembolic disease in adults, such as pulmonary embolus.

OCA Skin cancer, nystagmus, and strabismus. Most patients are registered blind.

P:

PKU Excellent if treatment commences within 2–3 weeks of life. If delayed, outcome is variable. If delayed till 6 months, some improvement in IQ occurs but likely to have moderate to severe learning disability.

Homocystinuria Good if treatment continues. Treatment prevents the development of complications but will not reverse damage that has already occured.

OCA Variable depending on the mutation.

Inborn errors of carbohydrate metabolism

D: Inherited biochemical disorders such as GSDs and galactosaemia that occur as a result of genetic mutations leading to disorders in the synthesis and degradation of carbohydrates.

A: **GSD:** a genetic mutation in any of the enzymes involved in the synthesis or degradation of glycogen. This → an abnormality in the quantity and/or quality of glycogen produced.
Galactosaemia: mutation → disorder of galactose metabolism with abnormally high plasma levels.

A/R: Family history, consanguinity.

E: **GSD:** 1/20 000–25 000 live births.
Galactosaemia: 1/30 000 (Ireland)–70 000 (UK) live births.

H: **GSD:** clinical manifestations vary widely from harmless to lethal.
Commonest Type Ia: presents at about 3–4 months with growth retardation, hepatomegaly, and hypoglycaemia. Other subtypes have varying degrees of myopathies.
Galactosaemia: neonates present with jaundice, vomiting, hypoglycaemia, and 2° convulsions. Later, may present with learning disability.

E: **GSD:** doll-like facies, short stature, hepatomegaly, protruding abdomen.
Galactosaemia: cataracts, hepatosplenomegaly, growth retardation, ascites.

P: **GSDs have been categorised:**
(1) Numerically in order of defect identification (Ia, Ib, II, III, IV, V, VI).
(2) According to organ involvement and clinical manifestation into liver and muscle glycogenoses.
Most common enzymatic defect is glucose-6-phosphatase deficiency (type Ia).
Galactosaemia: associated with 3 enzyme deficiencies: the most common enzyme deficiency 'classic galactosaemia' is galactose-1-phosphate uridyl transferase, which is an autosomal recessive genetic condition.

I: Definitive diagnosis requires demonstration of enzymatic defect in the affected tissue.
GSD: low glucose, elevated uric acid, lactate, and triglycerides are indicative.
Galactosaemia: screened for neonatally in some parts of the UK; reducing substances in the urine may be found in patients ingesting lactose.

M: **GSD:** aimed at maintaining normal blood glucose levels by continuous NG infusion of glucose initially until uncooked starches can be introduced into diet (slow release of glucose).
Galactosaemia: requires elimination of galactose from diet. Breast-feeding is contraindicated.

C: **GSD:** hepatic adenoma, renal disease (renal stones and hypertension).
Galactosaemia: ovarian failure, learning difficulties, developmental delay.

P: **GSD:** complications occur mainly in adults whose disease was not adequately treated during childhood. Long-term complications are avoided by good metabolic/dietary control.
Galactosaemia: if untreated, severe classical galactosaemia is a life-threatening disorder. Most patients reach adulthood if they follow a galactose-exclusion diet.

Inflammatory bowel disease

D: Chronic idiopathic inflammatory disorders of the bowel divided into:
UC: affects mucosa from the rectum to the terminal ileum.
CD: affects any area of the GI system.

A: **Genetic susceptibility:** high incidence in 1st degree relatives and ~50% concordance in monozygotic twins.
Environmental triggers: infections, seasonal variation, psychosocial factors (major life events).

A/R: Family history, smoking (only CD).

E: **UC incidence:** 10–15/100 000/yr. Peak in early adulthood.
CD incidence: 5–10/100 000/yr. Bimodal age distribution with the 1st peak beginning in late teens.

H: **UC:** more classical 'colitis' symptoms, ↑frequency of defaecation, rectal bleeding, abdominal cramps, urgency, anorexia, weight loss, fever.
CD: more insidious presentation often without presence of 'colitis' symptoms; anorexia, malaise, failure to thrive. May have abdominal pain (especially right lower quadrant possibly with mass), and ↑stool frequency.

E: Tachycardia, anaemia, digital clubbing, growth retardation. In Crohn's disease may have fissures, fistulae, and other perianal disease.

P: **UC: Macro:** affects the colon +/− backwash ileitis. Starts distally at the rectum and progresses proximally. *Lesion* is *continuous* with mucosal erythema, ulceration, and inflammatory pseudopolyps.
Micro: distortion of crypt architecture, inflammatory cell infiltrate, goblet cell depletion, and crypt abscesses.
CD: affects anywhere in the GI tract from mouth to anus. Consists of *segmental* disease with skip lesions, thickening (oedema or fibrosis) of mucosa, deep ulceration, fissuring or fistulae.
Micro: transmural inflammation, lymphoid aggregates, non-caseating granulomas.

I: **Bloods:** ↓Hb, ↑CRP, ↑ESR (good indicator of severity), serum folate, B_{12}, LFTs (abnormality requires investigation with ERCP, USS, biopsy for PSC).
UC: AXR; to exclude toxic megacolon. Colonoscopy with biopsy (except in acute episodes where phosphate enema and sigmoidoscopy are preferred).
CD: as in UC plus barium meal, OGD, small bowel follow-through to assess upper GI system.

M: **UC: Medical:** sulphasalazine and other 5-ASA compounds (oral or enema) are used long-term to reduce rate of relapse. ↑Doses of topical/oral corticosteroids if unresponsive.
Surgical: fulminant disease may require pancolectomy (curative).
CD: Dietary: high-fibre, low-fat, low-residue diet, with vitamin supplementation. In severe cases may use elemental diet.
Medical: sulphasalazine and other 5-ASA compounds or oral prednisolone for maintenance. Azathioprine and metronidazole in intractable disease.
Surgical: delay for as long as possible as inflammation can occur anywhere along the GI system. Reserved for intractable disease, fistulae, and fissures.

C: Erythema nodosum, episcleritis, renal stones, digital clubbing, sacroiliitis, arthralgia, pyoderma gangrenosum.
UC: toxic megacolon (intestinal dilation of >5.5 cm on AXR), perforation, colorectal carcinoma, PSC.
CD: megaloblastic anaemia, gallstones, perianal disease (tags, fissures, fistulae, purulent discharge), strictures, obstruction, failure to thrive.

P: **UC:** 20% relapse/year. Majority go on to full employment and have normal life expectancy.
CD: chronic disease with ↑morbidity. Extra-intestinal manifestations may be the major cause of morbidity. Most children still lead active, full lives with intermittent flare-ups.

Intraventricular haemorrhage (IVH)

D: Intracranial haemorrhage usually arising in the germinal matrix and periventricular regions of the brain.

A: The germinal matrix tissue is located adjacent to the lateral ventricles. It is the site of origin of migrating neuroblasts from the end of the first trimester and has become highly cellular and richly vascularised by 24–26 weeks. The vessels are thin-walled and fragile and susceptible to damage from fluctuations in cerebral blood flow leading to haemorrhage. Haemorrhage in this area may destroy the migrating neuroblasts and impair subsequent brain development. The germinal matrix involutes by the 36th gestational week which is why preterm infants are most affected.

A/R: **Factors that ↑/↓ BP:** hypovolaemia, hypotension, hypertension, pulmonary haemorrhage, mechanical ventilation, ↑pCO_2, ↓pO_2, prolonged labour, PDA.
Others: HIE, severe RDS, pneumothorax, coagulopathy.

E: **Commonest in very low-birth weight infants:** 30–40% of infants weighing < 1500 g; 50–60% of infants weighing < 1000 g.

H&E: Highest incidence in first 72 h of life, 60% within 24 h, 85% within 72 h, < 5% after 1 week postnatal age.
Signs and symptoms: seizures, poor tone, apnoea, lethargy.
Signs of raised ICP: bulging fontanelle, Cushing response (↑BP, ↓HR).
Monitor head circumference: for progressive hydrocephalus.

P: See **A**.

I: **USS is used in the diagnosis and classification of IVH:**

- Grade I: IVH in germinal matrix only.
- Grade II: IVH without ventricular dilatation.
- Grade III: IVH with ventricular dilatation.
- Grade IV: IVH with periventricular haemorrhagic infarct.

M: **Routine screening:** indicated in infants < 32 weeks gestational age within the 1st week of life and should be repeated in the 2nd week.
Prevention: maintain acid–base balance and avoid fluctuations in BP.
Supportive care: ventilatory support and blood transfusion in large haemorrhage.
Treatment of ↑ICP: diuretics (mannitol) and hyperventilation may be required.
Interventional: external ventriculostomy or permanent ventricular–peritoneal shunt.

C: Hydrocephalus (10–15%), neurological impairment.

P: **Grade I and grade II:** rarely have harmful neurological consequences, as they originate in the germinal matrix that disappears and do not normally extend into the white matter.
Grade III: 30–45% incidence of neurological impairment.
Grade IV: 60–80% incidence of neurological impairment.

D: Invagination of part of the intestine into itself.

A: The cause is unknown in most cases. May complicate viral infections such as otitis media, gastroenteritis, or URTIs; swollen Peyer's patches in the ileum may stimulate peristalsis causing an intussusception. In 2–10%, a lead point for the intussusception is found, i.e. inverted appendiceal stump, Meckel's diverticulum, an intestinal polyp, or adhesions from recent surgery.

A/R: HSP, CF patients are at risk if they become dehydrated.

E: 1–4/1000 births. M : F = 4 : 1. It is the most common cause of intestinal obstruction between 3 months and 6 years of age. 60% are <1 year, 80% occur before 2 years. Peak age 6–9 months. Rare in neonates.

H: **Classically present with a triad of symptoms:**
(1) Vomiting is the most common symptom; initially non-bilious and reflexive then becomes bilious.
(2) Colicky, severe, and intermittent pain associated with screaming and often pallor. The child is often reported to draw legs up to the abdomen; may appear well or lethargic in between episodes.
(3) Red currant jelly stools occur in only one-third of cases.

Note: may present with only lethargy and poor feeding.

E: **Abdomen:** soft and non-tender in early stages, but eventually abdomen becomes distended and tender. May find sausage-shaped mass in the right side of the abdomen or blood on rectal examination.

P: The most common site of invagination is the terminal ileum into the caecum. Constriction of the mesentery obstructs venous return, which → engorgement and oedema with subsequent bleeding. If the obstruction is not relieved, engorgement will prevent arterial perfusion that results in intestinal infarction and perforation.

I: **Bloods:** ↑WCC (late sign), ↑CRP, U&Es.
AXR: look for dilated small bowel and absence of gas in the region of the caecum.
Barium/air/water-soluble contrast enema: diagnostic and curative in 75% of children.

M: **Reduction is an emergency.**
Therapeutic enema: using barium, air, or water-soluble contrast, pressure can be gradually ↑ to force back the intussuscepting bowel. Therapeutic enemas, should only be used if the history is <24 h and if there is no evidence of peritonism or severe dehydration.
Surgical reduction: if therapeutic enema fails or is contraindicated.

C: Prolonged intussusception can → shock, peritonitis, and intestinal perforation. Overzealous reduction may rarely → perforation.

P: Untreated intussusception is almost always fatal within 2–5 days. Recovery is best if reduction occurs within 24 h of onset. The risk or recurrence is 10% with barium reduction and 2–5% with surgery.

Klinefelter syndrome

D: Genetic defect in the sex chromosomes in males which → a karyotype of 47XXY (80–90% of cases) or more rarely a mosaic of 46XY/47XXY.

A: **Common causes:**
(1) Extra X chromosome.
(2) Non-disjunction during meiosis and mitosis (50–60% due to maternal non-disjunction, and 75% due to meiosis I errors).
(3) Anaphase lag during meiosis and mitosis.
Rare causes: structural chromosomal abnormalities.

A/R: ↑Maternal age, paternal non-disjunction errors.

E: 1–2/1000 live-born males. It is the commonest cause of hypogonadism in males.

H&E: **Antenatal:** condition may be detected on chromosomal analysis.
Childhood: speech, language, and reading problem may be noted; however, most XXY individuals have normal intelligence.
Puberty: patients may lack 2° sexual characteristics because of a decrease in androgen production. This results in sparse facial/body/sexual hair, a high-pitched voice, a female type of fat distribution and ↓muscle mass. Small testes (< 2 cm) and gynaecomastia may also be noted due to elevated oestrogen levels and ↑oestrogen/testosterone ratio.
Adulthood: usually present with infertility or gynaecomastia. Also suffer from erectile dysfunction and low libido. Adults are usually tall, with disproportionately long arms and legs.

P: **Testicular biopsy:** seminiferous tubular hyalinisation, sclerosis, and atrophy with focal hyperplasia of mostly degenerated Leydig cells. Germ cells are markedly deficient or absent.

I: **Bloods:** elevated LH/FSH, ↓ testosterone.
Chromosomal studies: confirm diagnosis on karyotype analysis once suspected.
Semen analysis: performed to assess whether conception is possible using ICSI.
Testicular biopsy: for evaluation of infertility.
Bone mass density: osteoporosis may develop in 25% due to lack of sex hormone regulation on osteoblast/osteoclast activity in the bone.
Echo: assess for MVP.

M: **Hormonal treatment:** testosterone replacement via IM injections or skin patches; this should commence as patients enter puberty. This helps in developing 2° sexual characteristics; however, does not ↑fertility.
Surgical intervention: persistent gynaecomastia should be treated by mastectomy as this reduces the ↑risk of breast carcinoma.
Regular follow-up: needed to assess bone mass density via DEXA scans and monitor effect of treatment.
Psychosocial: support for patient in dealing with this lifelong condition.

C: (1) ↑Risk of breast cancer with gynaecomastia (∼20 × population risk).
(2) Osteoporosis and related fractures.
(3) Infertility is seen in practically all individuals with a 47XXY karyotype who require ICSI to reproduce. Patients with Klinefelter syndrome mosaicism (46XY/47XXY) may be fertile.
(4) MVP (50–60% of patients).

P: Individuals have a normal lifespan, and can lead relatively normal lives.

Legg–Calvé–Perthes disease (LCPD)

D: Avascular necrosis of the capital femoral epiphysis of the femoral head.

A: Idiopathic or 2° to DDH, sickle-cell crisis, SUFE, steroid use, and trauma.

A/R: DDH, achondroplasia, mucopolysaccharidosis, rickets.

E: 1/2000 children < 15 years. **Peak age:** 7 years; range: 2–12 years. **Sex:** M : F = 5 : 1. 10–15% of cases are bilateral.

H: **Wide range of presentation:**
(1) Hip or groin pain that may be referred to the knee or lateral thigh.
(2) Painless limp particularly after exertion.
(3) Pain in the anterior part of the thigh with an antalgic gait.
(4) Usually no history of trauma.

E: **Look:** atrophy of the quadriceps muscles 2° to disuse on the affected side, leg length inequality.
Feel: not so useful in examining the hip (hidden joint).
Move: restricted range of movement, particularly internal rotation and abduction.
Roll test: patient lies in a supine position. The examiner rolls the foot of the affected hip into internal and external rotation. This test invokes guarding or spasm, especially with internal rotation.

P: Rapid growth of the epiphysis of the femur during childhood may not be matched by equal growth in blood supply. This can → avascular necrosis of the proximal head of the femur. Revascularisation occurs, and new bone ossification starts. At this point, some children develop LCPD, while others continue to have normal bone growth and development. LCPD occurs when there is a subchondral fracture (smooth bone tissue beneath cartilage). This usually results from normal physical activity, not from traumatic injuries.

I: **Bloods:** FBC, CRP if suspicion of septic arthritis (fever, pain at rest).
Hip X-ray (frog leg views): 5 stages of disease:
(1) Cessation of growth at the capital femoral epiphysis; smaller femoral head epiphysis and widening of articular space on affected side.
(2) Subchondral fracture; linear radiolucency within the femoral head epiphysis.
(3) Resorption of bone.
(4) Re-ossification of new bone.
(5) Healed stage.

M: **Paediatric orthopaedic referral:**
(1) Rest the hip in the early irritable phase.
(2) Subsequently encourage movement of hip to overcome any stiffness.
(3) External splints or surgical osteotomy may be required to maintain hip in a position of internal rotation and abduction so as to reduce weight bearing.

C: May result in permanent femoral head deformity and early osteoarthritis.

P: Later onset (> 10 years) and degree of radiological involvement are associated with early osteoarthritis. Most children, however, have a favourable outcome.

Leukaemia, acute lymphoblastic (ALL)

D: Uncontrolled proliferation of a clone of immature lymphoid cells from a single abnormal cell. ALL is divided into B-cell (>80%), T-cell (15%) or mixed (2%) depending on what cell line the clone lies.

A: Lymphoblasts (arrested at an early stage of development) with varying cytogenetic abnormalities (gene mutations and chromosome translocations) undergo malignant transformation and proliferation with subsequent replacement of normal marrow elements, bone marrow failure, and infiltration into other tissues.

A/R: **Risk factors:** environmental (radiation, viruses).
Genetic associations: Down syndrome, Fanconi anaemia, achondroplasia, ataxia telangiectasia, xeroderma pigmentosum, X-linked agammaglobulinaemia, ↑risk in siblings.

E: Commonest malignancy of childhood (30% of all malignancies). 85% of childhood leukaemias are ALL. **Peak age:** 3–7 years, 2nd peak in old age.

H&E: **Symptoms of bone marrow failure:** anaemia (fatigue, dyspnoea), bleeding (spontaneous bruising, bleeding gums, and menorrhagia if adolescent), infections (bacterial/viral/fungal).
Symptoms of organ infiltration: meningeal involvement (headache, visual disturbance and nausea), cranial nerve palsies, retinal haemorrhage or papilloedema on fundoscopy, lymphadenopathy, tender bones, hepatosplenomegaly, testicular swelling, mediastinal compression in T-cell ALL (dyspnoea).

P: Malignant lymphoblasts are subclassified using FAB classification based on morphology (L_1–L_3).

I: **Bloods:** ↓Hb (normochromic, normocytic) +/− ↓platelets, ↑WCC, ↑uric acid, ↑LDH, clotting screen.
Bone marrow aspirate/trephine biopsy: hypercellular (> 30% lymphoblasts).
Immunophenotyping: uses antibodies to identify cell antigens in order to classify ALL cells into early B, common, pre-B, B cell, and T cell.
Cytogenetics: karyotype abnormalities such as chromosomal loss/gain, translocation, e.g. t(9, 22).
Cytochemical stains: B-lineage ALL stains positive with PAS stain, T-lineage ALL stains with acid phosphatase.
LP: CSF analysis for meningeal involvement.
CXR: mediastinal lymphadenopathy, thymic enlargement, lytic lesions.
Bone X-rays: 'punched-out' lesions of the bones, e.g. skull due to leukaemic infiltration.

M: **Combination cytotoxic chemotherapy:**
Remission induction: oral prednisolone, IV vincristine, IM/SC *L*-asparaginase (3–4 weeks).
Intensification or consolidation: addition of cytosine arabinoside, daunorubicin.
Prophylaxis of CNS involvement: intrathecal/IV methotrexate, cranial irradiation at 1 year in high-risk cases (WCC $> 50 \times 10^9$, age > 9 years, T cell, pre-B cell with t(1, 19)).
Maintenance chemotherapy: (2–3 years) 6-mercaptopurine (/day), methotrexate (/week), vincristine/prednisolone (/month), co-trimoxazole (*Pneumocystis carinii* prophylaxis).
Stem cell transplantation: only in children with t(9, 12), WCC $> 200 \times 10^9$, B cell with t(8, 14).
Supportive care: antiemetics, central venous access (Portacath/Hickman line) blood products/growth factors, infection treatment and prophylaxis, mouth care, counselling.

C: **2° to treatment:** tumour lysis syndrome (rapid cell death with initiation of chemotherapy may precipitate renal failure).
Long-term sequelae of chemotherapy: cardiotoxicity, fertility problems, 2° malignancy, (intracranial tumours, NHL), and relapse.

P: 70% 5-year survival.
Poor prognostic features: Philadelphia translocation t(9, 22); 0–15% disease-free at 5 years, age < 2 and > 10 years, males, WCC $> 100 \times 10^9$/L, t(4, 11), T-cell ALL, CNS involvement at presentation, lack of response to treatment.
Good prognostic features: t(12, 21).

Leukaemia, acute myeloblastic (AML)

D: Malignant clonal disease characterised by proliferation of myeloblasts in the bone marrow or blood.

A: Myeloblasts (arrested at an early stage of development) with varying cytogenetic abnormalities (gene mutations and chromosome translocations) undergo malignant transformation and proliferation with subsequent replacement of normal marrow elements, bone marrow failure, and infiltration into other tissues.

A/R: AML may be 1° or arise on a background of myeloproliferative or myelodysplastic disease or previous chemotherapy.
Occasionally associated with Sweet syndrome (acute febrile neutrophilic dermatitis), which also occurs in other malignant diseases.
Individuals with Down syndrome are at higher risk (some forms of AML are linked to chromosome 21).

E: Accounts for 15% of all childhood leukaemias.

H: **Symptoms of bone marrow failure:** anaemia (lethargy, dyspnoea), bleeding (DIC or thrombocytopenia in case of M_3 promyelocytic leukaemia), infections (bacterial/viral/fungal).
Symptoms of tissue infiltration: gum swelling/bleeding, CNS involvement (headaches, nausea, diplopia), bone pain.
Systemic symptoms: malaise, weakness, fever.

E: **Signs of bone marrow failure:** pallor, cardiac flow murmur, ecchymoses, and infections of the mouth (*Candida*, herpes simplex), skin (pseudomonas), respiratory system, perianal + perineal (*E. coli, streptococcus faecalis*) area.
Signs of tissue infiltration: skin rashes, gum hypertrophy, deposit of leukaemic blasts may rarely be seen in the eye ('chloroma'), hepatosplenomegaly, and lymphadenopathy.

P: **FAB classification into 8 morphological variants** (M_0–M_7).

I: **Bloods:** ↓Hb, ↓Plt, ↑↓WCC, ↑uric acid, ↑LDH, fibrinogen/D-dimers (if DIC is suspected in M_3).
Blood film: AML blasts show cytoplasmic granules or Auer rods.
Bone marrow aspirate/biopsy: hypercellular with $>30\%$ blasts.
Special: immunophenotyping and cytogenetics for FAB classification.

M: **More intensive than ALL as remission is more difficult to achieve and maintain.**
Emergency: DIC with M_3; requires FFP and platelet transfusions.
Chemotherapy: combination cytotoxic chemotherapy weekly, e.g. cytosine arabinoside, daunorubicin, etoposide (topoisomerase inhibitor) + all-*trans* retinoic acid with therapy for M_3 to induce differentiation.
Stem cell transplantation.
Supportive care: central venous access, (Portacath/Hickman line) blood products/growth factors, infection treatment and prophylaxis, mouth care, counselling.

C: **Leucostasis:** WBC thrombi, causing pulmonary or CNS infarcts, may occur if ↑↑WCC.
Sequelae of chemotherapy: infertility, cardiotoxicity, malignancy, tumour lysis syndrome (rapid cell death with initiation of chemotherapy, may precipitate renal failure).
Sequelae of BMT: GVHD, relapse, rejection.

P: 5-year survival > 50%
Poor prognostic features: WCC $>$ 100 000, $<$ 2 years at presentation.

D: Chronic disease of the hepatic cells → decrease in overall liver function.

A: (1) **Chronic active hepatitis:** autoimmune disease of parenchyma (autoimmune hepatitis) or biliary tree (primary sclerosing cholangitis), HBV, HCV, drugs (NSAIDs, antibiotics (nitrofurantoin), anticonvulsants, paracetamol (indirect)).
(2) **Wilson disease:** genetic disease of copper metabolism which → deposition of copper in the liver, brain, kidneys, and cornea.
(3) **CF** (see chapter).

A/R: Family history, developing countries (HBV/HCV).

E: **HBV:** 5% of the world's population has chronic HBV infection. Age at infection determines the rate of progression from acute infection to chronic infection; ~90% in the perinatal period, 20–50% in children aged 1–5 years, and < 5% in adults.
HCV: 1% worldwide chronic infection, with development of cirrhosis and hepatocellular carcinoma in a number of cases, after an interval of 10–15 years.
Autoimmune hepatitis: 0.1–1.2/100 000. M : F = 1 : 4. **Peak ages:** 10–20 years, 45–70 years.
Wilson disease: 1/30 000 live births.

H&E: **Presentation may be acute or insidious:**
General: failure to thrive, lethargy, loss of fat and muscle bulk.
GI: distended abdomen (ascites/hepatosplenomegaly), scrotal swelling, dilated abdominal veins (portal hypertension).

Autoimmune hepatitis: skin rash, lupus erythematosus, arthritis, haemolytic anaemia, or nephritis.
Wilson disease: Kayser–Fleischer rings in the corneas at > 7 years, neurological features > 12 years such as speech changes, tremor, difficulty with fine motor tasks and gait.

P: **HBV/HCV:** death of hepatocytes at an interface between parenchyma and connective tissue, with infiltration of plasma cells and lymphocytes.
Autoimmune hepatitis: inflammatory cell infiltrate with 'piecemeal' hepatocellular necrosis.
Wilson disease: autosomal recessive disorder with multiple mutations on chromosome 13 → a reduced synthesis of caeruloplasmin (copper-binding protein) and defective excretion of copper in bile.

I: **HBV/HCV:** serology and antigen screen.
Autoimmune hepatitis: hypergammaglobulinaemia (IgG > 20 g/L), positive autoantibodies (smooth muscle cell antibodies), antinuclear antibodies, liver/kidney microsomal antibodies.
Wilson disease: ↓serum caeruloplasmin, ↓serum copper, ↑urinary copper, ↑hepatic copper.

M: **HBV:** immunisation in at-risk infants. Supportive management + α-interferon.
HCV: α-interferon. No vaccine is available.
Autoimmune hepatitis: 90% of children respond to prednisolone and azathioprine.
Wilson disease: penicillamine reduces hepatic and CNS copper deposition, zinc reduces copper absorption, pyridoxine prevents peripheral neuropathy.
All may require liver transplantation in end-stage liver disease.

C: Coagulation defects, electrolyte disturbances, hypoglycaemia.

P: Depends on the underlying pathology. The prognosis is greatly improved with adequate and prompt treatment of the underlying condition. Autoimmune hepatitis has the best prognosis due to its high response to therapy.

Liver failure, acute

D: Acute failure of the hepatic cells to maintain normal function, also called fulminant hepatitis.

A: Acute liver failure is caused by damage to the hepatic cells by:

(1) **Infection:** acute viral hepatitis (A, B), EBV may precipitate infectious mononucleosis hepatitis.

(2) **Drugs/inadvertent poisoning:** paracetamol, isoniazid, halothane, and *Amanita phalloides* (poisonous mushrooms).

(3) **Reye's syndrome:** there is convincing evidence that aspirin given in patients <14 years of age is associated with an acute non-inflammatory encephalopathy with associated liver damage.

A/R: See **A**.

E: Uncommon in children. EBV is common in adolescents (age 15–20) as it is transmitted through exchange of bodily fluids of close contacts.

H&E: **General:** may present within hours with jaundice, encephalopathy, coagulopathy, hypoglycaemia or other electrolyte disturbances.

Encephalopathy:

(1) Young children: there may be a history of alternating periods of irritability and confusion with drowsiness.

(2) Older children may have a history of aggression and being unusually difficult.

P: **Reye's syndrome:** microvesicular fatty infiltration of the liver.

I: **Bloods:** ↑bilirubin (although may be normal in the early stages), deranged clotting, ↑↑transaminases, ↑ALP, ↑plasma ammonia, and ↓glucose.
ABG sampling: for frequently associated acid–base imbalance.
Viral serology: to detect hepatitis strain.
Radiology: CT brain in encephalopathy; may show cerebral oedema.
Other: EEG may show acute hepatic encephalopathy.

M: **Treatment of complications:**
Hypoglycaemia: dextrose infusion.
Sepsis: IV broad-spectrum antibiotics.
Coagulation defect: FFP and H_2-blockers/proton pump inhibitors to prevent gastric bleed. Vitamin K is avoided unless necessary as may mask deterioration in clotting factors, which is used as an indication for liver transplantation.
Cerebral oedema: fluid restriction and diuresis with mannitol.
Liver transplantation: with worsening clinical, biochemical, and clotting profile; prothrombin time is the best marker of liver failure.

C: Cerebral oedema, haemorrhage from gastritis or coagulopathy, sepsis, and pancreatitis.

P: Although acute liver failure is uncommon, it has a high mortality.
Poor prognostic signs:

(1) Liver starting to shrink in size.

(2) Rising bilirubin with falling transaminases.

(3) ↑Coagulation defect.

(4) Progression to encephalopathy and coma.

A patient who progresses to coma and does not receive a liver transplant has a 70% mortality.

Lymphoma, Hodgkin's

D: Lymphomas are neoplasms of lymphoid cells, originating in lymph nodes or other lymphoid tissues. Hodgkin's lymphoma is characterised histopathologically by the presence of the **Reed–Sternberg cell**, and T-cell dysfunction.

A: Likely to be due to environmental triggers in a genetically susceptible individual (may be due to defect in cell-mediated immunity). EBV genome has been detected in ~50% of Hodgkin's lymphomas, but its role in its pathogenesis is unclear.

A/R: Higher socio-economic groups. Past history of infectious mononucleosis.

E: **Incidence:** 1/100 000/year. Non-Hodgkin's (85%) > Hodgkin's (15%).
Age of presentation: late childhood/adolescence. M : F = 2 : 1.

H: **Enlarged lymph nodes:** painless enlarging mass, often in neck, occasionally axilla or groin.
Constitutional B symptoms: fevers > 38° C, night sweats, weight loss > 10% body weight in 6 months.
Others: pruritus, cough or dyspnoea with intrathoracic disease, SVC obstruction (blackouts, dyspnoea, feeling of *fullness* in the head).

E: (1) Non-tender firm lymphadenopathy (cervical, axillary, or inguinal).
(2) Splenomegaly, occasionally hepatomegaly.
(3) Skin excoriations.
(4) Signs of intrathoracic disease: SVC obstruction (facial oedema, ↑JVP).

P: **Histological subtypes:**
(1) Nodular sclerosing (70%).
(2) Mixed cellularity (20%).
(3) Lymphocyte-predominant (5%).
(4) Lymphocyte-depleted (5%).
Reed–Sternberg cell: large cell with abundant pale cytoplasm and 2 or more oval lobulated nuclei containing prominent 'owl-eye' eosinophilic nucleoli.

I: **Bloods:** ↓Hb (normochromic, normocytic) leucocytosis, eosinophilia, lymphopenia (with advanced disease), ↑ESR, ↑CRP, ↑LDH, ↑AST/ALT (with liver involvement).
Lymph node biopsy: immunophenotyping, cytogenetics.
Bone marrow aspirate and trephine biopsy: involvement seen only in very advanced disease.
Imaging: CXR, CT (thorax, abdomen, pelvis), gallium scan, PET scan.
Staging (Ann Arbor):
I: single lymph node region.
II: 2 or more lymph node regions on one side of the diaphragm.
III: lymph node regions involved on both sides of the diaphragm.
IV: extranodal involvement (liver or bone marrow).
A: without B symptoms; **B:** with B symptoms; **E:** localised extranodal extension;
S: spleen involved.

M: **Stage I, IIA:** radiotherapy; *mantle* for above the diaphragm, *inverted Y* for below the diaphragm (para-aortic lymph nodes and groin) +/− chemotherapy.
Stage III, IV: cyclical (×6) chemotherapy (ABVD) +/− radiotherapy.
Stem cell transplantation: for relapsed disease.

C: **Late malignancy 2° to chemotherapy:** AML (1% at 10 years), NHL, or solid tumours.
Inverted Y irradiation: infertility, early menopause, skin cancer.
Mantle irradiation: thyroid disease, accelerated CAD, pulmonary fibrosis.

P: **Stage I, II:** 80–90% cured. **Stage III, IV:** 50–70% cured.
Poor prognostic factors: B symptoms or if lymphocyte-depleted.

D: Lymphomas are neoplasms of lymphoid cells originating from lymph nodes or other lymphoid tissues. NHLs are a diverse group, 85% B-cell, 15% T-cell, and NK-cell neoplasms, ranging from indolent to aggressive disease, which can be referred to as low, intermediate, and high grade NHL.

A: Environmental triggers in a genetically susceptible individual results in DNA mutations or translocations → uncontrolled proliferation of lymphoid cells.

A/R: **Inherited or acquired immunodeficiency syndromes:**
(1) HIV and high-grade B-cell lymphomas.
(2) EBV and post-transplant lymphoproliferative disease.
(3) Prior treatment with chemo- or radiotherapy.
Infective causes:
(1) HTLV-1 → adult T-cell leukaemia/lymphoma.
(2) EBV → Burkitt's lymphoma.
(3) *Helicobacter pylori* → MALT lymphoma.

E: **Incidence:** 1/100 000/year. Non-Hodgkin's (85%) > Hodgkin's (15%).
Onset: late childhood/adolescence. M : F = 2 : 1.

H: **Localised:** Stage I, II, relatively unusual; cough, sore throat with enlarged neck glands or tonsils, or in the ileocaecal region presenting as intussusception.
Aggressive/rapidly enlarging:
(1) Mediastinal T-cell tumour: respiratory or SVC obstruction.
(2) Infiltrative, large retroperitoneal B-cell tumour: vomiting, abdominal pain.
(3) Dissemination (Stage IV): presents as ALL with masses.

E: **General:** non-tender, firm lymphadenopathy (cervical, axillary, or inguinal), hepatosplenomegaly, signs of bone marrow involvement (anaemia, infections, or purpura).
Specific:
Cutaneous T-cell lymphomas:
(1) Mycosis fungoides: well-defined, thickened, indurated, scaly, plaque-like lesions.
(2) Sézary syndrome: erythroderma, peripheral lymphadenopathy, and cellular infiltrates of atypical lymphocytes (Sézary cells).

P: REAL classification based on clinical, biological, and histological criteria.

I: **Bloods:** ↓Hb 2° to bone marrow involvement: neutropaenia and thrombocytopaenia (may also be due to hypersplenism), ↑ESR, ↑CRP, ↑LDH (used as a prognostic marker), ↑ALT/AST with liver involvement, ↑Ca^{2+}.
Blood film: lymphoma cells may be visible in some patients.
Lymph node biopsy: immunophenotyping, cytogenetics.
Bone marrow aspirate/biopsy.
Imaging: CXR, CT (thorax, abdomen, pelvis).
Staging: Ann Arbor (see Hodgkin's lymphoma) in NHL prognosis is more closely related to histological type (REAL classification).

M: **T-cell NHL:** chemotherapy and CNS prophylaxis as for ALL. There is improved prognosis in T-cell Stage III with the UK ALL X protocol giving a 90% 4-year survival.
B-cell NHL: aggressive pulsed chemotherapy regimen for Stage IV disease using alkylating agents and methotrexate is improving survival. Surgery is only indicated for emergency tumour obstruction of airways, bowel, or bladder.

C: **2° to treatment:** bone marrow suppression, nausea and vomiting, mucositis, infertility, tumour lysis syndrome, 2° malignancies.

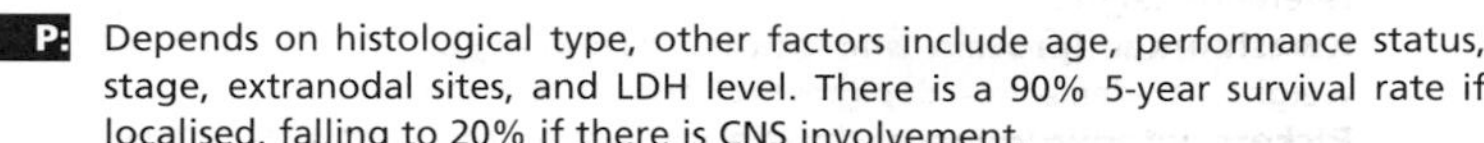

P: Depends on histological type, other factors include age, performance status, stage, extranodal sites, and LDH level. There is a 90% 5-year survival rate if localised, falling to 20% if there is CNS involvement.

D: **Weight < 80% of standard for age, using WHO growth charts.**
Marasmus (calorie deficiency): < 60% median reference weight for median reference height.
Kwashiorkor (protein and calorie deficiency): <80% median reference weight + oedema +/− depigmentation and hair changes.
Rickets: vitamin/mineral deficiency; clinical syndrome arising from under-mineralised bone matrix in growing bone due to lack of vitamin D, calcium, or phosphate.

A: **Malnutrition in developing countries:**
- **Environmental:** war, lack of transport, lack of infrastructure, market-based economy, drought.
- **Educational:** late weaning at > 12 months causes kwashiorkor with a subsequent high starch diet.
- **Physical:** chronic GI infection (hookworm, parasitic, protozoal), HIV, malaria, TB.

Malnutrition in developed countries:
- **Environmental:** poverty, parental neglect/abuse; Munchausen syndrome by proxy.
- **Educational:** unskilled feeding techniques in infants, nutritional deficiencies due to restrictive diets.
- **Physical:**
  (1) ↓ Reserve: preterm infants have reduced fat and protein reserves.
  (2) ↓ Ingestion: limitation by cleft palate abnormalities, anorexia induced by chronic disease.
  (3) Poor retention: GORD, pyloric stenosis.
  (4) Poor absorption: coeliac disease, CF, cow's milk protein intolerance.
  (5) ↑Metabolic rate: CF, infection, malignancy.
  Psychological: AN, emotional deprivation.

A/R: See **A**.

E: **Developing countries:** 15 million deaths/year from malnutrition and associated infections.

H: **Assessment of dietary intake:** food quantities, methods of food preparation, snacks, drinks, eating away from home (day care, relatives), budget limitations, who feeds the child? **Include a careful social history.**

E: Poor nutritional intake results first in weight loss, then decline in linear growth, then stunting of circumferential growth of head. Serial measurements are more useful than single measurements.
Marasmus: wasted, lethargic, no oedema.
Kwashiorkor: oedematous, flaky skin with depigmentation, protuberant abdomen, hepatomegaly, angular stomatitis, glossitis.
Rickets: bones are soft and long bones are easily deformed, thickened metaphyses.

P: See **D**.

I: **Bloods:** Hb, MCV, iron, folate, B_{12}, albumin.
Rickets: vitamin D level, Ca^{2+}, phosphate, ALP.
Radiology: wrist X-ray; cupping and fraying of metaphysial surfaces and widened epiphyseal plate in rickets.

M: **Developing countries:** community-based refeeding clinics are more effective than hospitalisation due to risk of nosocomial infections.

Refeeding:

(1) Manage dehydration and electrolyte deficiencies first (K^+, Ca^{2+}, phosphate, Mg^{2+}).
(2) Introduce feeding slowly to prevent electrolyte shifts and 2° lactose intolerance.
(3) Once full strength feed is tolerated introduce high-energy feeds.
(4) Treat infections/infestations.

Rickets: oral supplements of vitamin D. Exposure to sunlight.

C: ↓Immunity, delayed wound healing, ↓intellectual function, stunting of growth and development, permanent bone deformity in rickets.

P: Malnutrition in developing countries is responsible for 60% of deaths in children under 5 years of age. Those who survive are later predisposed to Type II DM and hypertension.

D: Non-rotation or incomplete rotation of the intestine around the SMA during embryological development, which predisposes towards intestinal obstruction and ischaemia.

A: During development normal rotation takes place in 3 stages around the SMA as the axis.
Non-rotation: arrest in development at stage 1 results in ↑risk for midgut volvulus.
Incomplete rotation: stage 2 arrest → incomplete rotation and is most likely to result in duodenal obstruction.

A/R: Gastroschisis, DDH, duodenal atresia, jejuno-ileal atresia, Hirschsprung disease, intussusception.

E: 1/500 live births. Commonest presentation in children is midgut volvulus.

H&E: 30–40% of patients with malrotation present within the 1st week of life, 50% by 1 month, and 75% by 1 year.
Acute midgut volvulus: usually presents < 1 year with sudden onset of bilious vomiting, abdominal distension, and severe infant colic.
Chronic midgut volvulus: recurrent abdominal pain and malabsorption syndrome. In between twisting episodes may appear normal.
Acute duodenal obstruction: usually presents in infancy with forceful vomiting, abdominal distension, and gastric waves. It is due to compression or kinking of the duodenum by peritoneal bands.
Chronic duodenal obstruction: usually presents in infancy to preschool age with bilious vomiting, failure to thrive and intermittent abdominal pain.
Internal herniation: patients have recurrent abdominal pain, which may progress from intermittent to constant. May develop vomiting or constipation.
Acute obstruction: tachycardia, abdominal distension, tinkling bowel sounds, vomiting.
Infarction/necrosis: shock, fever, and signs of acute peritonitis.

P: See **A**.

I: **Bloods:** ↑WCC, ↓Hb (microcytic anaemia with GI blood loss), U&E abnormal due to vomiting/abdominal secretions.
AXR: *Double bubble* sign of duodenal obstruction (produced by an enlarged stomach and proximal duodenum with little gas in the remainder of the bowel).
Barium meal/follow-through: the investigation of choice in stable patients to detect volvulus/obstruction.

M: **Pre-op management:** correction of fluid and electrolyte deficits, broad-spectrum antibiotics, NG tube to decompress proximal bowel.
Ladd procedure: reduction of volvulus (if present), division of mesenteric bands, placement of small bowel on the right and large bowel on the left of the abdomen, and appendicectomy.

C: Bowel strangulation, necrosis and perforation → septic shock.
Midgut volvulus: short bowel syndrome and malabsorption.
Surgical: wound infection, dehiscence, adhesions that may require re-operation.

P: Most forms of malrotation have a good outcome with prompt surgical intervention in a paediatric surgical department. In midgut volvulus, prognosis depends on how much bowel is preserved.

Marfan syndrome

D: Autosomal dominant inherited connective tissue disease.

A: Abnormal synthesis of extracellular matrix glycoprotein fibrillin is caused by mutations in fibrillin-1 gene on chromosome 15q21.1.
Dominant-negative mutation: abnormal gene is recessive, therefore some normal fibrillin is produced; however, mutant fibrillin-1 disrupts microfibril formation and results in destruction of normal fibrillin, thus giving an autosomal dominant picture.

A/R: 1st degree relatives affected.

E: 1/10 000 live births worldwide.

H&E: **General:** usually tall, thin individual with $\downarrow$upper/lower segment ratio and arm span $>$ height.
Musculoskeletal: muscle hypotonia, hyperextensible lax joints with frequent dislocation that $\rightarrow$ a delay in achievement of motor milestones.
Hands: arachnodactyly (long thin fingers), thumb sticks out of clenched hand (Steinberg sign).
Spine: scoliosis, kyphosis.
Feet: pes planus.
Eyes: loss of vision due to upward lens dislocation, myopia, retinal detachment.
Cardiovascular: may develop aortic root dilatation and AR (early diastolic murmur), MVP and MR (ejection click and pansystolic murmur), arrhythmias.
Respiratory: spontaneous pneumothoraces (SOB, pleuritic chest pain).
Skin: striae on shoulders, hips, and lower back.
Others: high-arched palate, pectus excavatum.

P: Electromicroscopic examination of fibrillin shows a significant $\uparrow$ in fraying of microfibrils. Fibrillin is a major building block of microfibrils, which are structural components of the suspensory ligament of the lens, elastin in the aorta, and other connective tissues.

I: **Molecular and genetic studies:** to confirm Marfan syndrome.
Imaging in aortic dissection:
(1) **CXR:** widened mediastinum, enlarged aorta/heart, apical blebs.
(2) **CT/MRI:** confirmation and extent of aortic dissection.
(3) **Echo:** to assess for aortic root dilatation, AR, MVP, and MR.
Slit lamp examination: to assess for lens dislocation.

M: **Multidisciplinary approach:**
Medical:
(1) β-blockers: delays aortic dilatation.
(2) Hormonal therapy for early induction of puberty to reduce ultimate height.
(3) Prophylactic antibiotics before bacteraemia-inducing procedures, e.g. dental, surgical.
Surgery: aortic aneurysm and dissection, AR and MR; patients require anticoagulants post-valvular surgery.
Ophthalmic: refractive lens for myopia, laser treatment for detached retina, removal of lens in some cases.
Orthopaedic: arch support for pes planus, surgery in severe cases of scoliosis/pectus excavatum.
Advice: avoidance of strenuous exercise and contact sports.
Genetic counselling.

C: Aortic dissection, bacterial endocarditis after surgery/dental treatment.

P: **Mortality:** if untreated, at 30–40 years of age, with good management many have a normal life expectancy. Cardiac problems are the commonest cause of death. Neonatal presentation is associated with a more severe course.

D: Infectious RNA viral illnesses.

A: **Measles:** transmitted by droplets or direct contact. Incubation period: 7–14 days. Infectious 2 days before symptoms and 4 days after onset of rash.
Mumps: transmitted by direct contact, droplet spread. Incubation period: 14–21 days. Infectious up to 7 days after the onset of parotid swelling.
Rubella: transmitted by droplet spread or via the placenta to the foetus. Incubation period: 14–21 days. Infectious 6–14 days after onset of rash.

A/R: Malnutrition, immunocompromise, not being immunised, contact with affected individuals.

E: **Measles:** 4/100 000; has dropped significantly from 800 000/year (1960s) to 3000/year (1990s) (UK figures) due to MMR vaccine.
Peak age: < 1 year (before immunisation) or older children not immunised. Commonest in developing countries.
Mumps: 3–4/100 000. **Peak age:** 5–9 years.
Rubella: 3–4/100 000. **Peak age:** > 15 years.

H&E: **Measles:** prodrome of fever, conjunctivitis, coryza, cough and Koplik's spots (grain-like white spots opposite lower molars and buccal mucosa). Rash appears 3–4 days later usually behind the ear and spreads to the whole body. Rash is initially maculopapular, but subsequently becomes blotchy and confluent. May desquamate in the 2nd week.
Mumps: up to 40% are asymptomatic. Prodrome of fever, muscular pain, headache, and malaise. Pain/swelling of one or both parotid glands.
Rubella: lymphadenopathy, malaise, fever, headache, coryza, maculopapular rash (small, pink) on face spreading within 24 h to chest, upper arms, abdomen, and thighs.

P: Entry is via the oropharynx with viral replication, viraemia, and subsequent involvement of glands and other tissues.
Measles: morbillivirus (paramyxovirus).
Mumps: paramyxovirus.
Rubella: rubivirus.

I: Usually a clinical diagnosis. Confirm by serology and/or viral culture.

M: **Supportive:** antipyrexials and encourage oral intake.
Medical: ribavirin may be used via SPAG for measles in the immunocompromised/high-risk infants.
Prevention of spread: MMR vaccine at 12–15 months with second dose at 4–6 years. Children should avoid school/day care until no longer infective.
Notification: measles, mumps and rubella are notifiable diseases (CCDC).

C: **Measles:** common; otitis media, pneumonia, diarrhoea, rare; encephalitis (1/5000), SSPE (1/100 000).
Mumps: viral meningitis (10%), encephalitis (1/5000), orchitis (more commonly affects adults), oophoritis, pancreatitis, deafness.
Rubella: arthropathy (common), encephalitis, thrombocytopenia, myocarditis, congenital rubella syndrome (75–90% transmission during 1st trimester).

P: **Measles:** mortality rate has fallen but still 750 000/year (UNICEF) usually due to pneumonia or diarrhoea (developing countries). Encephalitis has 15% mortality and results in seizures, deafness, hemiplegia, and severe learning difficulties in 40%. SSPE is a severe illness that may rarely affect children ~7 years after the initial illness.
Mumps: the disease is usually self-limiting and has a good prognosis.
Rubella: not a debilitating disease in adults. Congenital rubella syndrome, however, may → developmental delay, hearing impairment, CHD, neurological, ophthalmic and endocrinological complications.

Meckel's diverticulum

D: Outpouching of the ileum along the antimesenteric border, which usually measures 3–6 cm and is ~50–75 cm from the ileocaecal valve (depending on patient's age). At least 25% of diverticula removed surgically contain heterotopic tissue of the stomach (acid-secreting parietal cells), pancreas, or intestine.

A: Due to partial or incomplete involution of the vitelline duct during embryogenesis (see **P**).

A/R: **DD:** acute appendicitis.

E: Most common congenital GI anomaly occurring in 2–3% of all infants but is symptomatic in very few (1/3000). M : F = 3 : 1.

H&E: Most children are asymptomatic.
Intermittent painless rectal bleeding: may present within the first 2 years of life, but up to the 1st decade when there is ulceration of the mucosa due to acid.
Signs and symptoms of anaemia: lethargy, pallor, and failure to thrive.
Intussusception: may occur in older children and → partial or complete obstruction of the intestine.
Acute diverticulitis of the Meckel's diverticulum: characterised by localised abdominal pain and tenderness below or to the left of the umbilicus; often accompanied by vomiting and is similar to appendicitis except for location of the pain. May occur at any age.

P: During embryogenesis the vitelline duct runs between the terminal ileum, the umbilicus, and the yolk sack and usually regresses by week 7. Failure to atrophy can lead to a number of congenital abnormalities such as a remnant fibrous band running from the diverticulum to the umbilicus, an umbilical cyst, an ileo–umbilical fistula, or Meckel's diverticulum. Meckel's diverticulum is the most common of these abnormalities and is formed when the entire duct, except the portion to the ileum, is obliterated.

I: Diagnosis depends mainly on clinical presentation.
Bloods: ↓Hb, ↓MCV.
Stool sample: for obvious or occult blood.
Barium meal and follow-through: to assess for stricture or obstruction of the intestinal tract.
Radionucleotide scan: IV infusion of technetium 99m is taken up preferentially by the mucous-producing cells of the acid-secreting ectopic mucosa. Sensitivity is 50–90%.

M: **No intervention is required unless the patient is symptomatic.**
If patient presents with obstruction or a picture resembling appendicitis, the diagnosis is often made at surgery. Small, asymptomatic diverticula encountered incidentally at laparotomy need not be removed. Whenever a normal appendix is found during an exploration for appendicitis, Meckel's diverticulum should be suspected.

C: Intestinal obstruction may → perforation of bowel wall and peritonitis.
Torsion may → ischaemic and subsequently gangrenous bowel, which can be fatal.

P: There are usually no long-term problems after Meckel's diverticulum is resected. Many individuals are asymptomatic all their lives.

Meconium aspiration syndrome

D: Respiratory distress in the neonate caused by the passage of meconium (foetal bowel contents) stained amniotic fluid into the respiratory system.

A: Foetal distress may result in the passage of meconium *in utero* into the amniotic fluid (meconium-stained liquor). Foetal hypoxia results in the initiation of respiratory movements prior to birth (primitive gasping reflex) and meconium-stained fluid may be aspirated into the lungs causing obstruction and chemical pneumonitis.

A: Low birth weight, postmaturity, cord compression, placental insufficiency.

E: Meconium staining occurs in 10–15% of live births; of these, 1–9% experience meconium aspiration syndrome.

H&E: **Meconium aspiration:** foetal tachycardia, bradycardia, or absence of foetal accelerations on CTG *in utero* identifies a high-risk infant. At birth the neonate may exhibit signs of postmaturity with evidence of weight loss and heavily stained yellow nails, skin, and umbilical cord.

Respiratory distress in the newborn: diagnosed at birth or within 4 h; consists of tachypnoea, tachycardia, recession; intercostal/subcostal/sternal/substernal, nasal flaring, grunting, harsh diminished breath sounds, chest may have an overinflated appearance (2° to air trapping). In severe cases the neonate may become cyanosed.

P:

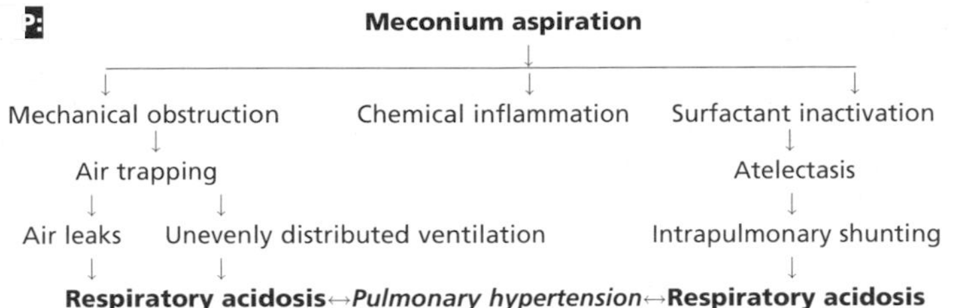

I: **CXR:** hyperinflation, flattening of the diaphragm, cardiomegaly, gross patchy shadowing.

ABG: ↓pO_2 occurs when there is right → left shunting of blood through the foramen ovale 2° to pulmonary hypertension.

M: Neonates born with meconium-stained liquor require a paediatrician to be present at birth.

Immediate assessment of the infant:

- If infant is vigorous and crying no further management is required, as visualisation of the airway and ET suctioning will not prevent aspiration.
- If the infant is floppy and not breathing, the airway should be suctioned under direct vision, either directly or via an ET tube/meconium aspirator.
- If at any stage during the resuscitation the HR falls bellow 60, oxygenation including intermittent PPV overrides the desire to clear the airway.

Subsequent management in NICU: antibiotics, ventilatory assistance, and exogenous surfactant therapy. Inhalation of NO and ECMO may be required.

C: Pulmonary hypertension (see separate chapter), pneumothorax.

P: Ultimate prognosis depends on the extent of asphyxial insult to the neonate *in utero*, and degree of meconium aspiration.

Meningitis

D: Infection of the subarachnoid space associated with an inflammatory response of the meninges.

A: **Bacterial:**
Neonatal to 2 months:
GBS, *gram-negative bacilli,* e.g. *Escherichia coli, Listeria monocytogenes.*
1 month to 6 years:
Neisseria meningitidis (meningococcus), *Streptococcus pneumoniae,* Hib.
> 6 years:
N. meningitidis, S. pneumoniae, mumps (pre-MMR).
Mycobacterium tuberculosis: can cause TB meningitis at all ages. Commonest in children aged 6 months to 6 years.
Viral: enteroviruses (80%), CMV, arbovirus. HSV is more likely to cause encephalitis (see chapter).

A/R: **Impaired immunity:** young age, defects of complement system (meningococcal susceptibility), splenic defect from sickle-cell disease or asplenia (*S. pneumoniae* and Hib susceptibility).
Factors associated with low socio-economic status: crowding, poverty and close contact with affected individuals (transmission by respiratory secretions).

E: **Varies in different countries:** UK 5.4–5.9% Republic of Ireland 10.5%, France 0.7%, Germany 1.3%.

- *N. meningitidis* (meningococcus) causes majority of bacterial infections in > 2 months. Has ↓ since the introduction of vaccine Men. C.
- *S. pneumoniae* (pneumococcal) meningitis is rising in incidence. Majority occur in < 2 years.
- Hib meningitis has fallen significantly since the introduction of the Hib vaccination.
- TB meningitis: rare; 161 cases documented in the UK in 2001.
- Enteroviruses have seasonal variation and are more common in autumn and summer.

H: **Prodromal features of infection:** otitis media/respiratory/GI symptoms.
Neonates: nonspecific symptoms such as fever (or hypothermia in severe illness), irritability, lethargy, seizures, shrill cry, or poor feeding.
Infants and children: fever, headache, neck stiffness, alteration in consciousness (from lethargy to coma), nausea, vomiting, photophobia, anorexia, rash, or seizures.

E: **Neck stiffness:** from meningeal irritation that prevents neck flexion.
Kernig's sign: in the supine position extension of leg is painful when knee and hip are flexed.
Rash: purpuric or petechial rash (usually non-blanching but may be blanching in initial stages of disease). Characteristic of meningococcal infection.
Signs of raised ICP: papilloedema, ↓level of consciousness, focal neurology (e.g. 6th nerve palsy), Cushing reflex (↑BP, ↓HR), decerebrate posturing.

P: Bacteraemia precedes infection and bacteria enter the CSF via the choroid plexus and rapidly multiply as local complement and antibody levels are low. Inflammation follows with disruption of the blood–brain barrier, oedema, and neutrophil infiltration.

I: **Bloods:** ↑WBC, ↑CRP, U&E, glucose, clotting studies, group and save.
Microscopy, culture and sensitivity: blood, stool, throat swab, urine, rapid antigen screen.

CT scan: if suggestive of ↑ICP to avoid coning on LP.
LP for CSF: contraindicated if focal neurological signs or ↑ICP suspected.
CSF in bacterial meningitis: neutrophils, ↑protein (1–5 g/L), ↓glucose (< 50% serum level).
CSF in viral meningitis: lymphocytes (initially neutrophils), normal/mildly elevated protein, normal glucose, PCR for diagnosis.
CSF: microscopy (Gram stain, e.g. for acid-fast bacilli in TB meningitis), culture and sensitivity.

M: **Start empirical parenteral antibiotic treatment before the results of investigations as meningococcal septicaemia is often rapidly fatal.**
Bacterial meningitis:

- 3rd generation cephalosporin: ceftriaxone or cefotaxime IV.
- Resistant *S. pneumoniae* is becoming more prevalent worldwide, but almost all strains in the UK are sensitive to third generation cephalosporins. Therefore routine use of vancomycin for community acquired meningitis is not justified in the UK.
- In infants < 3 months ampicillin should be started empirically to cover for *L. monocytogenes*.
- TB meningitis requires 6–9 months therapy with isoniazid, rifampicin, pyrazinamide and streptomycin.

Culture and sensitivity will indicate subsequent antibiotic therapy.
Corticosteroids: studies of patients with Hib meningitis have shown some improvement in morbidity (deafness or neurological deficit) with corticosteroid treatment alongside antibiotics. Data is lacking in pneumococcal and meningococcal meningitis.
Supportive care: analgesics, antipyretics.
Notification: meningitis is a notifiable disease (CCDC).
Contact prophylaxis: 2/7 of rifampicin for meningococcal infection.
Immunisations: BCG, men C, Hib.
Prevention: there are effective vaccines against *N. meningitides* C and *A*. Pharmaceutical companies are developing a combination vaccine containing B and C conjugate vaccines; this vaccine will prevent more than 90% of cases of meningococcal meningitis in Europe.

C: **During illness:** convulsions, cerebral oedema, circulatory shock, DIC.
Neurological sequelae: hearing loss (10%), therefore all children must have audiometry testing ~ 2/3 weeks after infection is treated, visual impairment, cerebral palsy, vasculitis may cause cranial nerve palsies, subdural effusions that usually resolve spontaneously, hydrocephalus, cerebral abscess, learning disability. All children must have neurological follow-up to enable early detection and management of these complications.

P: **Bacterial:** overall mortality 5–10%; neurological complications 10–20%.

- Meningococcal meningitis: mortality 7–20%, with septicaemia 18–53%, usually have favourable neurological outcome if they survive the acute illness.
- Pneumococcal meningitis: has a lower mortality than meningococcal meningitis but ↑ association with adverse neurological sequelae.
- TB meningitis: 15–30% of those affected do not survive, and up to 25% of people who recover may have long-term neurological sequelae.

Viral: 95% have complete recovery with no neurological sequelae.

Mesenteric adenitis

D: Inflammation of the mesenteric lymph nodes, with systemic illness and abdominal symptoms.

A: **Virul URTIs:** the commonest cause of mesenteric adenitis.
Bacterial URTIs: 2° to group A β-haemolytic streptococcus.
GI: *Yersinia enterocolitica* (commonest bacterial cause), *Helicobacter jejuni*, *Campylobacter jejuni*, and *Salmonella* or *Shigella* species.

A/R: Most common DD for acute appendicitis.

E: Affects children of all ages.

H: Mesenteric adenitis is often a diagnosis of exclusion; however, may be a positive diagnosis if a patient undergoes an unnecessary laparotomy for suspected appendicitis.
Recent infectious injury: URTI or GI infection; symptoms of coryza, pharyngitis, or gastroenteritis may still be present (mainly diarrhoea).
GI: vague abdominal pain may vary intermittently.

E: **Signs of acute appendicitis:**

- excessive vomiting
- significant anorexia
- usually low-grade fever
- periumbilical region/RIF tenderness
- pain becomes continuous
- fixed tenderness in RIF
- once peritoneum is involved guarding and rebound tenderness
- localised tenderness of anterior rectal wall
- unusual to have signs of URTI.

Signs of mesenteric adenitis:

- little vomiting
- mild anorexia
- may have high fever
- periumbilical region/RIF tenderness may also be present
- pain is intermittent
- tenderness shifts depending on the position of the child
- no true signs of peritonism
- no localised tenderness on rectal examination
- often have signs of URTI.

P: **Macro:** enlargement of mesenteric lymph nodes.
Micro: proliferation of B and T cells 2° to infectious process.

I: **Bloods:** ↑WCC, U&E (may be dehydrated), ↑CRP.
USS of RIF: to visualise appendix and exclude acute appendicitis.

M: **Careful observation:**

- Admit for regular reassessment to differentiate between mesenteric adenitis and acute appendicitis.
- Persisting local tenderness in the RIF lasting more than 3–6 h warrants surgical exploration.

C: None.

P: Mesenteric adenitis is a benign self-limiting disease.

D: Autosomal dominant multisystem disorder characterised by progressive muscle wasting, muscle weakness, and myotonia (abnormal sustained contraction of muscle).

A: **Genetic defect:** caused by expansion of CTG nucleotide triplet repeats at the 3′UTR of the myotonic dystrophy gene on chromosome 19. This gene codes for DMPK.
Genetic anticipation: the disease has earlier onset or ↑severity in the offspring than in parents as a result of further triplet repeat expansion in successive generations.

A/R: Family history, antenatal history; polyhydramnios.

E: 2/10 000 live births. Severe congenital type is much rarer and almost always inherited via the mother.

H: **Depends on number of CTG repeats:**
(1) **Unaffected individuals** (5–27 repeats).
(2) **Mild myotonic dystrophy** (50–100 repeats): cataracts, slight muscle weakness in adulthood.
(3) **Classical myotonic dystrophy** (100–1000 repeats): myotonia, muscle wasting, frontal balding, hypogonadism, cardiomyopathy, cardiac arrhythmias, DM, respiratory impairment, adverse reactions to anaesthesia.
(4) **Congenital myotonic dystrophy** (1000–4000 repeats).
- **At birth:** hypotonia, respiratory and feeding difficulties, marked facial weakness. Myotonia is not a feature of the condition at this stage.
- **If infant survives:** gradual improvement in muscle strength and tone, delayed motor development, persistence of facial weakness, severe learning disability (60–70% of cases), classic features of myotonic dystrophy by the age of 10.

E: **Peripheral weakness:** hands (unable to release grip), forearms, and feet as opposed to proximal weakness (hip, shoulder) in other dystrophies.
Myopathic facies: facial muscle weakness and wasting; bilateral ptosis, wasting of frontalis and temporalis, and weakness of sternomastoids; all of which result in lack of facial expression.

P: Disturbance in muscle fibre maturation with incomplete differentiation.
Infants: small undifferentiated muscle fibres.
Children: type 1 fibre atrophy; central nuclei, sarcoplasmic masses, ring fibres.

I: **Bloods:** CPK may be raised. **Muscle biopsy:** see **P**.
EMG: characteristic 'diver bomber' spontaneous electrical discharge by age 3.
DNA mutation analysis: sizing of the repeat array by PCR and/or Southern blotting.

M: **Multidisciplinary approach:**
Medical: myotonia may be treated with quinine or procainamide. Support respiratory and GI problems. Monitor for deformities.
Surgical: cataract operations.
Orthopaedic: ankle–foot arthroses for footdrop.
Occupational therapy: specially designed utensils for hand weakness.
Genetic counselling: for antenatal diagnosis.
Psychological support: for parent and child.

C: Joint contractures, foot deformities, early onset dementia.

P: Depends on the number of CTG repeats, extent of learning disability, and early appropriate multidisciplinary involvement. The older the child is when muscle weakness is first noticed, the slower the progression and less serious the consequences. Most do not survive past 50 years of age.

Near-drowning

D: **Drowning:** death from asphyxia <24 h of submersion in water.
Near-drowning: survival >24 h after submersion episode.

A: 2° **causes:** seizures, head or spine trauma, cardiac arrhythmias, alcohol/drug ingestion, syncope, apnoea, suicide, hypoglycaemia.
$<$ **1 year:** bathtubs/buckets of water. Consider child abuse in all cases.
1–5 years: residential swimming pools.
15–19 years: ponds, lakes, rivers, and oceans.

A/R: Inability to swim, failure to observe water safety rules, unsupervised swimming.

E: **UK incidence:** 0.8/100 000/year; 54 children died of drowning in 2000.
Worldwide: $\frac{1}{2}$ million died of drowning in 1998 (BMJ).
Peak age: toddlers <4 years of age and 15–19 years. M : F = 12 : 1 boating injuries, M : F = 4 : 1 non-boating injuries, bathtubs F $>$ M.

H: Most patients are found after having been submerged in water for an unobserved period. Relevant factors in the history include time under water, associated trauma, drug/alcohol use, water contamination, water temperature, rescue manoeuvres, response to resuscitation.

E: Hypothermia, tachycardia, bradycardia, tachypnoeia, ↓GCS. Severe cases may result in cardiorespiratory arrest.

P: Following submersion in water, 90% aspirate water or gastric contents (wet drowning), 10% develop laryngospasm (dry drowning). In both cases resultant hypoxia and metabolic acidosis can affect:
CNS: hypoxic neuronal injury and subsequent cerebral oedema.
Cardiovascular: cardiac dysrhythmias +/− myocardial damage that may → cardiogenic shock and hypovolaemia 2° to ↑capillary permeability and intracompartmental fluid shifts.
Respiratory: aspiration causes disruption of surfactant, pulmonary oedema, and may result in ARDS.
The **mammalian diving reflex** is protective and occurs if suddenly immersed in cold water. It produces apnoea, bradycardia, and vasoconstriction of nonessential vascular beds with shunting of blood to the coronary and cerebral circulation.

I: **Bloods:** ABG, FBC, U&E, LFTs, drug/alcohol screen, blood cultures.
Monitoring: cardiac, pulsoximetry.
Trauma series: cervical spine/chest/pelvic X-ray.
CT head: if deteriorating GCS/focal neurology.

M: Rescue and basic life support at the scene are the most important factors in determining outcome. Transfer to emergency department.
Airways: cervical spine immobilisation, consider ET intubation, NG tube to prevent vomiting.
Breathing: 100% O_2 via reservoir bag. Consider mechanical ventilation if poor respiratory effort, altered GCS, severe hypoxia, severe acidosis, or significant respiratory distress.
Circulation: fluid resuscitation +/− inotropes if BP not responsive, catheterisation, central venous access.
Disability: AVPU (initial assessment), GCS (full assessment of neurological disability).
Exposure: consider spinal injuries in all diving accidents. Correct hypothermia as may exacerbate bradycardia, acidosis, and hypoxaemia. Remove wet/cold clothing, external warming (bear-hugger, radiant lamp), active care rewarming if temperature $<32^\circ$C (warmed IV fluids, ventilator gases, gastric/bladder lavage, peritoneal lavage). Resuscitation should not be discontinued until core temperature $>32^\circ$C.

Prevention: adult supervision, fencing around swimming pools, basic life support education in the community.

C: ARDS, acute renal/hepatic failure, DIC.

P: 70% of children survive if basic life support is provided at the waterside. Only 40% survive without early basic life support despite hospital measures. Of those who survive ~30% result in some degree of neurological impairment. **Prognostic factors:** immersion time, time to first gasp, core temperature (< 33°C is protective), acidosis, hypoxia. No implication whether salt or fresh water immersion.

Necrotising enterocolitis (NEC)

D: Severe GI disease that occurs in the first few weeks of life.

A: **Hypoxic-ischaemic injury:**

(1) NEC is associated with hypotension, hypothermia, hypoxia, anaemia, PDA, indomethacin therapy, and umbilical vessel catheterisation.
(2) There is a strong association with placental function as measured by the antenatal end diastolic flow in the umbilical artery.
(3) Intestinal injury may be related to absent or reduced ability of the neonatal intestine to regulate blood flow and oxygenation in the gut.

Enteral feeding:

(1) NEC is virtually never seen until infant is enterally fed.
(2) There is ↑risk of ischaemia as nutrient absorption ↑ oxygen demand, induces possible GI dysmotility and stasis.
(3) Breast milk is protective against the development of NEC.
(4) There is a particular association between hyperosmolar formula feeds and NEC.

Infectious disease:

(1) Bacterial proliferation plays an important role in NEC, but it is not known if it is a 1° initiator of the disease.
(2) Micro-organism involvement is indicated by the tendency for NEC to be epidemic.

A/R: Preterm infants, low birth weight.

E: NEC accounts for 1–5% of all NICU admissions.

H: Onset can be either insidious with feeding difficulties or sudden with peritonitis, septic shock, or death.

E: Findings depend on the severity of NEC:
Systemic: lethargy, temperature instability, or jaundice.
Respiratory: apnoea or respiratory distress.
CV: hypotension, poor perfusion or pallor.
GI: abdominal distension and tenderness, ↑gastric aspirates, bilious vomiting, bloody stools.

P: **Hypothesis:** neonates have an immature immune system and mesenteric vascular control. GI dysmotility or stasis plus an ↑ metabolic demand of the intestines can give rise to bacterial overgrowth and/or ischaemic stress. Tissue hypoxia proceeds to mucosal injury and the invasion of bacteria into the damaged mucosa.

I: **Bloods:** FBC, clotting screen, U&E. **Cultures:** blood, stool.
AXR: early signs are thickening of the bowel wall and abnormal gas patterns. This progresses to intramural gas, and in severe cases gas may be seen in the portal blood system. Signs of intestinal perforation.

M: Aggressive treatment should be started on recognition or suspicion of NEC.
General: fluid resuscitation and correction of electrolyte disturbances.
Feeding: stop enteral feeding for 2 weeks and replace with TPN. Refeeding should start with breast milk where possible.
Infection: broad-spectrum IV antibiotics.
Surgery: up to one-third of infants require resection for necrotic/perforated bowel.

C: Strictures, fistulae, abscess formation, recurrent NEC, 'short gut' syndrome, malabsorption, cholestasis, and enterocyst formation.

P: NEC is the commonest cause of death in neonates undergoing surgery. Mortality is 30–40% in this group.

D: Excess amount of bilirubin in the neonatal circulation gives rise to yellow discoloration of the skin and sclera.

A: **Physiological unconjugated hyperbilirubinaemia:** due to the following neonatal factors:

(1) Instability of foetal Hb: neonates have ↑RBC volume but ↓RBC survival.
(2) Defective bilirubin metabolism: immature hepatic function results in defective hepatic uptake of bilirubin and defective bilirubin conjugation.
(3) Defective bilirubin excretion: neonates have absent gut flora.

Breast milk jaundice: a physiological prolonged unconjugated hyperbilirubinaemia that peaks in the 2nd week and resolves very slowly (up to 3 months). It is thought to be due to a factor in breast milk that inhibits UDPGA glucuronyl transferase resulting in a prolonged unconjugated hyperbilirubinaemia.

Unconjugated haemolytic hyperbilirubinaemia in neonates:

(1) Immune-mediated: haemolytic disease of the newborn that may be due to ABO or Rh incompatibility.
(2) Hereditary: spherocytosis, elliptocytosis, G6PD deficiency, pyruvate kinase deficiency.
(3) Acquired: congenital infection, bacterial sepsis.

Unconjugated non-haemolytic hyperbilirubinaemia in neonates:

(1) ↑Hb load; haemorrhage, polycythaemia.
(2) Galactosaemia, hypothyroidism.
(3) Crigler–Najjar syndrome: complete absence of UDP glucuronyl transferase in the liver.
(4) Gilbert's syndrome: mild deficiency of UDP glucuronyl transferase.

Conjugated hyperbilirubinaemia in neonates:

(1) Infection: HAV, HBC, HCV, CMV, rubella, herpes simplex.
(2) Metabolic: CF, galactosaemia.
(3) Intrahepatic: congenital hepatic fibrosis.
(4) Extrahepatic: biliary atresia, choledochal cyst.
(5) Toxic: TPN-related, UTI, drugs.
(6) Endocrine: hypopituitarism, hypothyroidism.
(7) Dubin–Johnson syndrome (↓ability to transport organic anions such as bilirubin glucuronide into biliary tree).
(8) Rotor syndrome: deficiency in organic anion uptake as well as excretion.

A/R: History of a previous sibling with jaundice, preterm infants, breastfeeding.

E: Affects 50% of all neonates; 33% of breastfed neonates have persistent jaundice after 2 weeks.

H: **General presentation:** may be entirely well in physiological jaundice, or unwell; vomiting, lethargy, poor feeding, behavioural changes, tachypnoea, instability of temperature, pale stools, and dark urine.

Age of onset: important in determining likely pathological cause.

< 24 h = pathological.

> 24 h = probably physiological (but beware sepsis/galactosaemia).

> 2 weeks = requires investigation.

E: Neonates become clinically jaundiced when the bilirubin level reaches 80–120 μmol/L. There is correlation between the level to which the jaundice extends and the serum bilirubin level. Because of variation in skin colour, the best place to look for jaundice in all infants is the sclera. Examine also for pallor, hepatosplenomegaly, signs of sepsis, and petechiae.

P: See **A**.

I: **Early jaundice (< 24 h):** FBC, reticulocyte count (↑ in haemolysis), blood film, maternal and infant ABO and Rh typing, direct Coomb's (antiglobulin) test, infection screen (blood cultures, TORCH screen).

Jaundice at >24 h: if normal history and examination, monitor only.
Persistent jaundice (>2 weeks): total serum bilirubin and conjugated fraction should be obtained. TFTs, LFTs, urine for reducing agents in G6PD, direct Coomb's (antiglobulin) test.
Conjugated hyperbilirubinaemia: requires urgent investigation; USS biliary tree +/− liver biopsy isotope scanning HIDA/DISIDA and referral to a paediatric liver centre.

M: **Treat the cause:** if jaundice is 2° to disease process.
Treatment of jaundice: independent of disease process if bilirubin levels are high or are ↑ rapidly to prevent bilirubin encephalopathy (kernicterus).
Intensive phototherapy: involves placing the neonate under a series of 450 nm wavelength lights on a radiant warmer bed. This converts the stereoisomer and makes it soluble so that it is excreted by the kidney. Masks should be placed over the neonate's eyes for protection.
Exchange transfusion: used if intensive phototherapy fails to lower bilirubin level, or in conjunction with phototherapy with extremely elevated bilirubin levels. All neonates with bilirubin levels over the 'exchange transfusion level' should have hearing screened.

C: Bilirubin is neurotoxic and previously caused seizures, dyskinetic (athetoid) cerebral palsy, sensorineural deafness, and learning disability.

P: Good with physiological jaundice as this usually resolves without the need for treatment and does not predispose the neonate to further episodes of jaundice in later life. In other causes prognosis depends on early identification and appropriate management.

D: Characterised by hypoalbuminaemia, proteinuria, oedema.

A: All causes of GN can result in nephrotic syndrome.

A/R: Sickle-cell disease, Alport syndrome (haematuric nephritis and sensorineural deafness), HIV.

E: **Developed countries:** minimal change GN is the cause of nephrotic syndrome in 90% of cases; commonest in boys < 5 years. Peak age: 2–4 years.
Developing countries: infectious causes of GN: malaria (40%), HBV infection (6%) and group A β-haemolytic streptococcal infection (rare).

H&E: **General:** anorexia, lethargy, oliguria, check BP.
GI: diarrhoea, poor feeding, abdominal pain.
Oedema: swelling of face, ascites, dependent oedema of legs/scrotum.
Symptoms of complications: infections, renal vein thrombosis, loin pain, haematuria.

P: **Proteinuria:** structural damage to the glomerular membrane and reduction of its negatively charged components prevents the action of repelling negatively charged proteins, which are therefore excreted in excess.
Hypoalbuminaemia: mediated by proteinuria and ↑breakdown of albumin in the kidney.
Oedema: due to ↓intravascular colloid osmotic pressure.

I: **Bloods:** U&E, ↓albumin, ↑ESR/CRP, lipid profile (2° hyperlipidaemia).
Post-infectious nephropathy: *Plasmodium falciparum* (thick and thin blood films), HBV (serology), group A β-haemolytic streptococcal infection (ASOT).
Urine dipstick: 3/4 + protein, microscopic haematuria.
MSU: microscopy, culture and sensitivity.
24 h urine collection: creatinine clearance and 24-h protein excretion.
Renal USS: other renal diseases may cause proteinuria, e.g. polycystic kidney disease.
Renal biopsy: reserved for older children with haematuria, ↑BP, ↑urea, and in children who do not respond to steroid treatment (10%).
Doppler USS, renal angiogram, CT, MRI: if renal thrombosis is suspected.

M: **Symptomatic treatment:** limit oedema with protein-controlled, low-sodium diet and diuretics in severe cases.
Monitor: BP, U&E, Ca^{2+}, weight, fluid balance.
Treatment of initial presentation: prednisolone; controlled trials have demonstrated that longer duration (6 months) of initial prednisolone treatment is associated with fewer relapses and lower total prednisolone dose over the first 2 years.
Treatment of relapse: prednisolone daily until in remission, then a slow gradual reduction of dosage.
Treatment of steroid-resistant patients: alternate day prednisolone with long-term cyclosporin + enalapril to treat hypertension.
Steroid-sensitive patients (85–90% cases) respond after 4 weeks, steroid-resistant (10–15% cases) have no remission after 4 weeks.
Prevention of complications: antibiotic cover (penicillin) whilst oedematous to prevent pneumococcal peritonitis and septicaemia, avoid prolonged bed-rest to prevent thrombosis.

C: **Renal failure:** due to hypovolaemia, especially following diuretics or due to renal vein thrombosis.
↑Susceptibility to infection: peritonitis, pneumococcal infections due to loss of Ig in the urine.
Hypercoagulability: renal vein thrombosis and DVT due to hypovolaemia, loss of antithrombin III and protein C and S in the urine, and ↑synthesis of fibrinogen in the liver, immobility 2° to leg oedema, steroid therapy.

Hyperlipidaemia: ↑synthesis of triglycerides and cholesterol with albumin in the liver.

Before the introduction of steroids, 60% of children with the relapsing form of nephrotic syndrome died. Steroids have revolutionised the prognosis of this condition; however, prognosis is affected by complications of the condition or treatment (S/E: steroids/immunosuppression).

D: An aggressive tumour originating in the neural crest cells that give rise to the sympathetic nervous system.

A: **Not known.**
Genetic association: found in siblings and identical twins.
Microscopic nodules of neuroblasts are found in foetuses of 17–20 weeks gestation. Genetic predisposition or environmental factors may prevent regression.

A/R: NF, Beckwith–Wiedemann syndrome (exomphalos, macroglossia, gigantism).

E: **Prevalence:** 10/million population.

H: **General:** weight loss, abdominal pain, fatigue, and vomiting.
Abdominal 1°(two-thirds of cases): abdominal mass as incidental finding by carer.
Pelvic 1°: chronic diarrhoea or ↑urinary frequency.
Olfactory 1°: unilateral epistaxis.
Metastases to bone: bone pain, limp, and pathological fractures.
Metabolic disturbances: sweating, pallor, diarrhoea, ↑BP due to catecholamine secretion.

E: **Abdominal 1°:** firm irregular non-tender mass, with metastases to the liver – ascites and hepatomegaly.
Olfactory 1°: mass in the nasal cavity, occlusion of nasal passageways, posterior extension may cause spinal cord compression → paraplegia and Horner syndrome.
Skin: SC nodules may be seen in infants; non-tender, bluish, and mobile.
Opsoclonus–myoclonus (2% of cases): progressive cerebellar ataxia, titubation of head, myoclonic jerks and chaotic conjugated eye movements, progressive mental regression.

P: Tumours are formed from uniform small, round cells with scanty cytoplasm and hyperchromic nuclei, forming nests within the fibrovascular matrix.
Staging:
I – confined to 1° organ.
II – tumour does not cross midline, possible ipsilateral lymph node involvement.
III – tumour crosses midline, possible bilateral lymph node involvement.
IV – distant lymph node and tissue involvement.
IV-S – as I or II but metastases confined to liver, marrow, and skin, with no bony metastases.

I: **Bloods:** ↓Hb, ↓MCV, serum ferritin, LFTs, U&E, coagulation screen, LDH.
Urine assay: for urinary catecholamines.
Imaging: AXR, CXR, CT, skeletal survey for osteolytic lesions, separation of cranial sutures.
Histology: bone marrow aspirate, biopsy/excision of lymph node or liver in disseminated disease for definitive diagnosis.

M: **Localised tumour:** surgical excision.
Disseminated disease (majority): chemotherapy is main-line therapy; radiation therapy for symptom relief or size reduction. BMT.

C: Complications of surgery, chemotherapy and radiotherapy.

P: **Prognostic factors:** tumour stage, age (inversely proportional; those < 1 year usually undergo remission), histopathology, molecular biology (↑ risk with N-myc amplification, 1p deletion), biochemistry (↑ risk with ↑ serum ferritin, ↑ LDH). Stage IV-S occuring in infancy has 85% regression rate.

Neurocutaneous syndromes

D: Disorders involving ectodermal tissue that cause defects in the skin and neurological system.

A: Autosomal dominant transmission 50%, *de novo* mutation 50%.
NF1 (von Recklinghausen disease): mutation on chromosome 17 that codes for tumour suppressor protein called neurofibromin.
NF2 (acoustic neuroma): mutation on chromosome 22.
TS1: mutation on chromosome 9 that codes for tumour suppressor protein called hamartin.
TS2: mutation on chromosome 16 that produces tumour suppressor protein called tuberin.

A/R: Family history (1st degree relatives).

E: **NF:** 1/4000 live births, **NF1:** 80%, **NF2:** 20%. **TS:** 1/6000 live births.

H&E: **NF1 + 2:** café-au-lait spots; well-circumscribed brown/cream lesions; six or more with >5 mm diameter in prepubertal patients and >15 mm in postpubertal patients, also axillary or inguinal freckling.
NF1:
Skin: two or more neurofibromata (nodules) distributed over peripheral nerves and cranial nerves, focal neurological deficit may occur due to nerve compression 2° to neurofibromata within a foramen.
Eyes: Lisch nodules; iris hamartomas; dome-shaped, clear yellow/brown lesions.
Bone lesions: sphenoid dysplasia (thinning of long bone cortex, long bone bowing), pseudoarthrosis.
NF2: deafness/tinnitus, headaches, possibly facial weakness and cerebellar ataxia, few cutaneous lesions.
TS:
Skin: depigmented 'ash-leaf' lesions that are fluorescent under UV light (Wood's light), acne-like rash; 'adenoma sebaceum' in butterfly distribution over bridge of the nose and cheeks, periungual fibromata, Shagrean patch.
Developmental delay: moderate to severe learning disability.
Neurological: infantile spasms, epilepsy.
Renal: renal angiolipomatas; flank pain, haematuria, hypertension.
Other: cardiac rhabdomyomata, retinal hamartomas.

P: **NF1:** neurofibromata are well-differentiated tumours consisting of elongated spindle-shaped cells and pleomorphic fibroblast-like cells.
NF2: bilateral tumours of the VIII cranial nerve. The tumours cause pressure damage to neighbouring nerves.
TS: multisystem involvement of small benign 'tuber-like growths' of connective tissue that grow in the brain and on other vital organs such as the kidneys, heart, eyes, lungs, and skin.

I: **NF1:** slit lamp examination for Lisch nodules. **MRI/CT brain:** glial nodules.
X-rays: pseudoarthrosis, scoliosis. **Skull X-ray:** 'Railroad track' calcification.
TS: urine analysis (haematuria), echo (cardiac rhabdomyomata), ECG (arrhythmias), MRI brain (tumours).

M: **Multidisciplinary approach: NF1 + 2:**
Paediatric: regular follow-up including BP monitoring, ophthalmology assessment, regular testing of VIII nerve, skeletal and cutaneous examinations for early recognition of complications.
Surgical: laser removal of nodules, orthopaedic or neurosurgical intervention.
TS: anti-epileptic medications, antihypertensives, neurosurgical intervention.
Antenatal diagnosis: amniocentesis/CVS.
Supportive/educational: TS patients often require special school attendance, emotional support for parents.

C: **NF1:** gliomas (benign, occasionally sarcomatous), scoliosis, spinal cord tumours, phaeochromocytoma, pulmonary hypertension, renal artery stenosis.
NF2: meningiomas, neurofibroma, Schwannoma.
TS: cardiac rhabdomyomas may cause hydrops foetalis, renal cysts, brain tumours; cortical tubers, subependymal nodules, giant-cell astrocytomas.

P: **NF1:** most just have café-au-lait spots with no neurological symptoms and live healthy long lives. Lifespan may be reduced by complications.
NF2: depends on complications, higher morbidity and mortality than NF1.
TS: depends on the severity of symptoms, learning disability, epilepsy, and renal/CNS complications.

Nocturnal enuresis

D: The involuntary passage of urine during sleep after the age of 5.
1° nocturnal enuresis (80%): never-achieved night-time dryness.
2° nocturnal enuresis: recurrence of bedwetting, having been dry for > 1 year.

A: **Developmental:** immature bladder control, with more frequent passage by day and night.
Environmental: stress, family break-up, maternal separation, moving house, birth of a younger sibling, hospital attendance.
Abuse: sexual, physical, emotional.
Structural: ↓bladder capacity, congenital anomalies.
Medical: UTI, constipation, epilepsy, occult spinabifida, DM/diabetes insipidus.

A/R: Familial, learning disability, large families, institutional upbringing.

E: 10% of 5-year-olds, 5% of 10-year-olds, 1% of 18-year-olds. M : F = 2 : 1.

H: **General assessment:** will the child ask for the toilet, dress/undress when needed? Is there a family history of enuresis? What is the attitude of the parents and child? What have they tried?
Medical assessment: are there any symptoms of frequency or burning on urination? Is there any incontinence during the day or faecal incontinence? This should alert you to underlying renal or neurological problems.
Social assessment: family stresses? Indication of sexual abuse?

E: **Neurological:** including sensation of saddle area.
Spine: for signs of occult spina bifida; hairy/pigmented patch.
Genital: for signs of abuse. **BP:** hypertension.

P: See **A**.

I: **Urine:** microscopy, culture and sensitivity.

M: **Supportive:** parental and child encouragement is the most important factor as success depends on their motivation. Stress importance of non-punitive approach.
Behavioural incentives: star charts for dry nights; 20–30% response.
Enuresis alarms: triggered when urine touches the sensor; 70–90% response, low relapse rate (10%).
Medication: used as a last resort in the older child.
Desmopressin (synthetic antidiuretic hormone):
- Intranasal or oral before bedtime.
- Poor long-term success rate, high relapse rate.
- Used for short-term control in special situations, e.g. sleepovers/camps.
- S/E: headache, runny nose, and nose bleeds.

Imipramine (rarely used):
- Presumed to work by relaxation of the bladder muscle and inducing a deeper sleep.
- Low initial and long-term cure rate, high relapse rate.
- Potentially fatal in inadvertent overdose due to cardiac arrhythmias.

Oxybutinin (antimuscarinic + direct relaxant urinary smooth muscle)
- Should be restricted to those children with a clear history of detrusor instability (daytime urgency, frequency, urge incontinence).
- S/E: Dry mouth, constipation, blurred vision.

C: Low self-esteem, depression, exasperation of parent which may → abuse, complications of organic causes of enuresis.

P: 'Cure' without treatment occurs in 15% per year. Nearly all children with 1° nocturnal enuresis will be cured with single or combination therapy (behavioural +/− alarms +/− medication). However, 1% of adults still suffer from nocturnal enuresis and need to be maintained on drug therapy. Children with 2° causes of enuresis require specific treatment of the underlying pathology or supportive management if this is not possible.

Obesity in children

D: BMI > 95th centile for sex and age.

A: Obesity is a disorder of energy balance that is usually multifactorial.
Diet: important factor not only in quantitative terms but also for relative fat/sugar content.
Psychosocial: lifestyle, poor physical activity, food preferences, personal and familial structure and stability.
Genetic predisposition: leptin deficiency (obesity, hyperphagia, and insulin resistance).
Genetic syndromes:
(1) **Prader–Willi syndrome:** compulsive eating, central fat distribution, hypogonadism, learning disability.
(2) **Lawrence–Moon–Biedl syndrome:** hypogonadism, moderate–severe learning disability.
(3) **Muscular dystrophy:** late presentation (see chapter).
(4) **Turner syndrome.**
Acquired syndromes: Cushing syndrome.

A/R: Obese parents or siblings (nature and/or nurture); obese families have obese pets, maternal DM.

E: 20% of children in the UK and USA are now overweight. 11% of 6-year-olds and 17% of 15-year-olds were obese in 1996 in the UK. Underlying disease only accounts for 5% of cases.

H&E: Dietary history, details of physical activities, psychosocial history. Screen for potential complications, in addition for specific syndromes associated with obesity. Detailed examination for stigmata of disease.

P: **Leptin deficiency:** leptin conveys a signal from adipose tissue to hypothalamic nuclei that integrate whole body fuel metabolism, informing those nuclei about the magnitude of fuel reserves. In the absence of leptin, the brain perceives energy availability as insufficient and therefore activates powerful mechanisms to restore fuel depots.

I: **Nutritional assessment:** BMI (wt (kg)/ht^2 (m)), triceps skinfold thickness.
Bloods: cholesterol level, triglyceride level. Endocrine assays for specific conditions, e.g. adrenal disease.
Urine: glucosuria (Type II DM).
Radiology: USS for specific conditions (ovaries, hepatic), CT/MRI head for specific syndromes.

M: Early intervention is important; requires good motivation from parent and child. Therapeutic aims include:
(1) Gradual reduction of excessive weight (growth needs should be taken into account).
(2) Dietary counselling with vitamin and micronutrient supplementation.
(3) Behaviour modification.
(4) Stepwise physical activity programme.
(5) Adherence to the plan requires strong support for the child and family.
Severe or complicated obesity: requires a protein-sparing very low-calorie liquid diet.

C: **Psychosocial:** peer discrimination, bullying, social isolation.
Growth: advanced bone age, children who are tall with ↑BMI are usually 2° to diet and physical inactivity, children who are short with ↑BMI are more likely to have organic cause/syndrome.
Respiratory: sleep apnoea, pickwickian syndrome (obesity–hypoventilation syndrome).
Orthopaedic: SUFE, Blount disease (idiopathic varus bowing of tibia).

Metabolic syndrome X: characterised by insulin resistance and atherogenic dyslipidaemia 2° to ↑triglycerides/↓HDL cholesterol and hypertension.
Endocrine: POS, precocious puberty.
Others: hepatic steatosis, gallstones.

P: Children with BMI > 95th centile are likely to be obese in adulthood. Patients with metabolic syndrome X are at significant risk of plaque build-up in arterial walls → coronary heart disease, stroke, aneurysm formation, and Type II DM.

Osgood–Schlatter disease

D: An extra-articular knee condition due to detachment of cartilage from the tibial tuberosity.

A: Stress and trauma to the tibial tuberosity 2° to overuse of the quadriceps muscle → the development of microfractures at the site where the tibial tuberosity inserts into the distal diaphysis.

A/R: Sports involving large amounts of running or jumping.
DD: tibial fracture, underlying tumour, quadriceps tendon avulsion, chondromalacia patellae, osteomyelitis of the proximal tibia, patellar tendonitis.

E: The most common knee disorder in adolescence; usually presents after adolescents have had their growth spurt: girls 10–11 years, boys 13–14 years.
M > F most probably due to ↑sporting activities in boys.
The disease is bilateral in up to 25% of cases.

H: Pain just below the knee where the patellar tendon inserts, usually for several months before presentation. There may be a memorable history of trauma. Pain is exacerbated by running, jumping, ascending and descending stairs, and relieved by rest.

E: **Principles of examining the knee:**
Look: soft tissue swelling over the proximal tibial tuberosity.
Feel: tenderness over the proximal tibial tuberosity at the site of patellar insertion.
Move: pain is reproducible on extending the knee against resistance, stressing the quadriceps, or squatting with the knee in full flexion.
Knee joint examination is normal as this is an extra-articular condition.

P: During periods of rapid growth, the force of contractions from the quadriceps muscles is transmitted through the patellar tendon onto a small portion of the partially developed tibial tuberosity. In Osgood–Schlatter disease, this results in microfractures through the ossification centre. Eventually, 2° heterotopic bone formation occurs in the tendon near the insertion of the tibial tuberosity and produces a visible lump.

I: **X-ray knee:** shows fractures of the tibial tubercle, possibly a separate ossicle.

M: **Rest:** avoidance of offending activity and other sports which strain the quadriceps (jumping, running).
Medical: NSAIDs may be given for pain relief and to reduce inflammation.
Orthopaedic devices: infrapatellar strap and in severe cases a knee immobiliser splint may be used.
Surgical: excision of the mobile ossicle is occasionally required.
Rehabilitation: quadriceps stretching and hip extension exercising should be advised after the acute symptoms have resolved so as to reduce tension on the tibial tubercle.

C: Non-union of the tibial tubercle, patellar tendon avulsion, continuing pain, bony prominence.

P: Most cases resolve spontaneously. Sometimes this condition may persist over a few months and these children require intervention or immobilisation of the knee joint. Some children may have problems with kneeling in adulthood.

D: Inflammation of the middle ear chamber.

A: **URT viruses (65%):**
(1) Rhinovirus (50%).
(2) RSV (13%).
(3) Influenza, parainfluenza, enteroviruses, and adenovirus (2%).
Bacteria (35%):
(1) *Streptococcus pneumoniae* (30%).
(2) Nontypeable *Haemophilus influenzae* (i.e. not Hib) (20%).
(3) *Moraxella catarrhalis* (20%).

A/R: **Environmental:** ↑exposure (nursery attendance), low–birth weight infants, parental smoking.
Mechanical: obstruction of Eustachian tube 2° to adenoidal hypertrophy, cleft palate, Down syndrome.

E: **Extremely common condition:** 2/3 children affected by 3 years, $\frac{1}{3}$ children will have 3 or more episodes. M > F.
Peak age: 6 months to 3 years, declines after 6 years.

H: Ear pain (infants may scream and pull at ear) preceded by URTI, fever, irritability, hearing loss. In infants, anorexia, vomiting, and diarrhoea may be the only presenting features.

E: On otoscopy the tympanic membrane is bright red and bulging with loss of normal light reflex. Occasionally, acute perforation occurs and pus is visible in the external auditory canal.

P: Initial hyperaemia of the tympanic membrane followed by serous fluid exuding into the middle ear that may later become purulent. The drum then looks dull and bulges. In uncomplicated infections the fluid becomes serous again and finally resolves.

I: Diagnosis is on otoscopic findings, but swab can be taken if there is discharge from the ear for microscopy, culture and sensitivity.

M: **At presentation:**
(1) Paracetamol (antipyretic and analgesic), decongestants are of unproven value.
(2) Amoxicillin; 5% of *Haemophilus* strains are resistant but sensitive to co-trimoxazole.
(3) Myringotomy; rarely, when very painful bulging drums need incision.
Prophylaxis: pneumococcal vaccine is not very effective in preventing otitis media. Nontypeable *H. influenzae* vaccine is in progress but less progress has been made for *M. catarrhalis*. The concept of a tribacterial vaccine remains to be tested in animal models.

C: **Chronic secretory otitis media/glue ear:** may be caused by recurrent infections and is the most common cause of conductive hearing loss in children. However, not all children with glue ear have hearing loss. Studies have shown that 70% of 4-year-olds, 20% of 5-year-olds, and 1% of 7-year-olds have glue ear, and not all of them have conductive hearing loss.
Persistent earache: may result due to pressure changes from obstruction to the Eustachian tube. If fluid persists for >4 months, grommets are inserted, with or without adenoidectomy if these are causing obstruction to the Eustachian tube.
Severe complications: mastoiditis, meningitis, subdural, extradural, or brain abcesses (rare).

P: Most cases resolve satisfactorily even if perforation occurs.

Patent ductus arteriosus (PDA)

D: Failure of closure or reopening of the ductus arteriosus after birth. In normal foetal circulation the ductus arteriosus is needed to allow blood to bypass the lungs.

A: **Preterm infants:** duct closure is delayed.
Full-term infants: there may be a defect in the constrictor muscles of the duct that may reopen with hypoxia or excess fluid administration.

A/R: Maternal rubella infection in the first 4 weeks of pregnancy.

E: **Preterm infants:** up to 40% in < 1500 g.
Full-term infants: 1/2000 live births. M : F = 1 : 2.

H: Variable depending on the size of the lesion and the coincident left → right shunting of blood through the pulmonary circulation.
(1) **Small defect:** asymptomatic.
(2) **Medium defect:** ↓exercise tolerance, left → right shunt may be associated with LRTIs, atelectasis, or pneumonia.
(3) **Large defect:** symptoms of CHF with dyspnoea and failure to thrive. Apnoea and bradycardia in neonates.

E: **Small defect:** normal pulses, continuous *machinery* murmur and thrill below left clavicle due to pressure gradient between aorta and PA throughout cardiac cycle, loud S_2 when both components close together.
Medium defect: wide pulse pressure, bounding peripheral pulses, may have signs consistent with LRTI.
Large defect: absent thrill, murmur present in systole only as pressures in the aorta and PA are equal in diastole, loud and single S_2, collapsing pulse.
Signs of CHF: tachycardia, tachypnoea, respiratory distress, displaced apex, cool peripheries. Measure BP.

P: **Pathophysiology of development of pulmonary hypertension:** ↑PA pressures due to left → right shunt eventually produce endothelial and muscular changes in the pulmonary vessel walls and → resistance to pulmonary blood flow that may be irreversible and will preclude definitive repair.

I: **CXR:** cardiomegaly, prominence of ventricles, ↑pulmonary vasculature.
ECG: usually normal; may have left atrial and ventricular hypertrophy.
Doppler echo: confirms patency and direction of flow.

M: **Preterm infants:** duct will usually close spontaneously; however, if symptomatic treatment is with fluid restriction, a prostaglandin inhibitor (such as indomethacin) or surgical ligation.
Older children: even asymptomatic small PDAs should be treated to prevent the lifelong risk of endocarditis. This is usually achieved by cardiac catheterisation (transvenous occlusion with a coil).

C: **Preterm infants:** IVH, intractable heart failure, CLD of prematurity.
Older children: infective endocarditis, pulmonary hypertension, Eisenmenger syndrome, pulmonary or systemic emboli.

P: If left untreated, the mortality rate is 20% by age 20 years, 40% by age 40 years, and 60% by age 60 years. Only an estimated 0.6% per year undergo spontaneous closure. Following PDA closure, patients experience no further symptoms and have no further cardiac sequelae.

D: Persistently raised pulmonary vascular resistance which → shunting of blood away from the lungs via the ductus arteriosus and foramen ovale.

A: After birth pulmonary vascular resistance normally declines rapidly as a consequence of vasodilation due to gas filling the lungs, a rise in postnatal PaO_2, a reduction in $PaCO_2$, and a rise in pH. 3 main mechanisms → failure or compromise of pulmonary vessel vasodilation.

(1) **Maladaptation of the pulmonary circulation due to injury:** this → an abnormal response to the lungs being filled with gas for the first time.
(2) **Chronic foetal hypoxia:** causes PA constriction via leucotriene activation.
(3) **Obstruction of the vasculature:** 2° to polycythaemia.

Specific causes: birth asphyxia, meconium aspiration pneumonia, group B streptococcal sepsis (release of prostaglandins), hypoglycaemia and maternal DM, pulmonary hypoplasia due to diaphragmatic hernia or oligohydramnios, capillary alveolar dysplasia.

A/R: Meconium-stained amniotic fluid, IUGR, foetal distress, Down syndrome.

E: 1/500–700 live births; occurs in term and preterm infants.

H&E: Should be suspected in all infants with cyanosis with or without foetal distress. Hypoxia is universal in all causes of PPH and does not respond to 100% O_2 (hyperoxia test).

Signs of respiratory distress: tachypnoea, recession: intercostal/subcostal/sternal/substernal, nasal flaring and cyanosis (common).

Signs of cardiogenic shock: may occur 2° to myocardial ischaemia and papillary muscle dysfunction with mitral and tricuspid regurgitation; presents with signs of ↓end-organ perfusion; oliguria, lethargy, hypotension.

P: See **A**.

I: **Bloods:** ABG, Hb, WCC, blood glucose.

CXR: oligaemic lungs.

Echo: to exclude CHD and extent of right → left shunt through patent foramen ovale.

M: **Antenatal:** at-risk infants should be identified in the antenatal period. Correct any predisposing conditions (hypoglycaemia and polycythaemia).

Ventilation: required in all neonates with PPH; tight control of pH, PaO_2, $paCO_2$. Can achieve better gas exchange with HFO ventilation.

Dilatation of pulmonary vasculature: requires invasive BP monitoring and support with all forms of vasodilator therapy.

- **Inhaled NO:** technically still under investigation but is still generally seen as the drug of choice.
- **Prostacyclin infusion:** when NO is not available.
- **Tolazoline:** nonselective α-adrenergic antagonist can be used as an adjunct to dilate the pulmonary vasculature.

Metabolic acidosis: Correction of acidosis causes pulmonary vasodilatation and improves cardiac output as acidosis has a negatively inotropic effect.

ECMO: a very effective rescue strategy for those who fail other treatments.

C: HIE.

P: With appropriate treatment complications are avoided and prognosis is usually the same as that of the underlying pathology.

Pneumonia

D: Infection of the lung parenchyma.

A: **Neonates:** organisms from the female genital tract: group B haemolytic streptococcus, *Escherichia coli* and gram-negative bacilli, *Chlamydia trachomatis*.

Infants–preschool children:

- **Viral (commonest):** parainfluenza, influenza, adenovirus, and RSV. RSV can be particularly dangerous to ex-preterm infants and infants with underlying CLD of prematurity.
- **Bacterial:** *Streptococcus pneumoniae* (90% of bacterial pneumonia). *Staphylococcus aureus* is uncommon but causes severe infection.

Older children–adolescents: as above, but also atypical organisms such as *Mycoplasma pneumonia* and *Chlamydia pneumoniae*. TB should be considered at any age.

Aspiration pneumonia: enteric gram-negative bacteria +/− *Strep. pneumoniae, Staph. aureus.*

Underimmunised: *Haemophilus influenzae*, *Bordetella pertussis*, measles.

Immunocompromised:

- **Viral:** CMV, VZV, HSV, measles, and adenoviruses.
- **Bacterial:** *Pneumocystis carinii*, TB.

A/R: **CLD:** Ex-preterm, CF, sickle-cell disease.

Immunocompromise: inherited (hypogammaglobulinaemia) or acquired (HIV, steroids).

Congenital cardiac abnormality: especially with large left → right intracardiac shunt.

Chronic aspiration: cerebral palsy, TOF, GORD.

Kartagener syndrome: ciliary dysfunction, bronchiectasis and dextrocardia.

E: Common, especially in the winter months.

H&E: **General:** fever, tachycardia, tachypnoea, cough, sputum (yellow, green, or rusty in *S. pneumoniae*), vomiting particularly post-coughing, poor feeding, diarrhoea, and preceding URTI (especially viral infections).

Signs of consolidation: ↓breath sounds, dullness to percussion, ↑tactile/vocal fremitus, bronchial breathing, course crepitations.

P: **Stages of lobar pneumonia:**

(1) Congestion with vascular engorgement, intra-alveolar bacteria.
(2) Red hepatisation: alveolar spaces fill with neutrophils, fibrin, and RBCs.
(3) Grey hepatisation: RBC disintegrates with fibrin and suppurative inflammation.
(4) Resolution: exudate in alveolar spaces is degraded and removed by macrophages.

Bronchopneumonia:

Macro: patchy areas of consolidation with grey/yellowish appearance.

Micro: neutrophil inflammatory infiltrate in bronchi, bronchioles, and adjacent alveoli.

I: **CXR:** focal consolidation suggests a bacterial cause; diffuse consolidation bronchopneumonia suggests a viral cause.

Bloods: ↑WCC if bacterial, ↑ESR/CRP, U&Es (SIADH).

Microscopy, culture and sensitivity: blood, sputum.

Blood film: RBC agglutination by *Mycoplasma* (cold agglutinins, see Haemolytic anaemia).

Immunofluorescence/PCR: can detect RSV on nasopharyngeal aspirate.

M: **Supportive treatment:** maintain $pO_2 > 8$ kPa, IV resuscitation in dehydration or shock.
Antibiotics: determined by presentation, i.e. viral/bacterial aetiology, severity, and CXR appearance; normally oral amoxicillin or erythromycin. If severe, IV cefuroxime +/− erythromycin, metronidazole for aspiration pneumonia.
Respiratory failure: CPAP/BiPAP, may require PICU transfer.
Immunisation: Hib (all infants), influenza and pneumococcal (at-risk infants).

C: Pleural effusion, empyema, lung abscess, septic shock, ARDS, ARF.

P: Most resolve within 1–3 weeks; however, children with an underlying respiratory, cardiac, immune or neurological abnormality may respond more slowly to treatment, and have a higher mortality.

Pneumothorax

D: Extrapulmonary extravasation of air into the pleural cavity.

A: **Pneumothorax:** usually caused by overinflation resulting in alveolar rupture. It may be spontaneous, idiopathic, or 2° to underlying pulmonary disease, trauma, or aspiration.
Tension pneumothorax: develops if the accumulation of air in the pleural space is sufficient to raise the intrapleural pressure above atmospheric pressure. A unilateral tension pneumothorax causes impaired ventilation in the collapsed affected side and impaired ventilation in the normal side due to mediastinal shift.

A/R: Vigorous resuscitation at birth, RDS, meconium aspiration syndrome, pulmonary hypoplasia, assisted ventilation therapy, asthma, pneumonia with empyema, CF, Marfan syndrome (2° to bullae).

E: **Spontaneous pneumothorax:** 1–2% of all live births. 10% are bilateral. M > F. Term/post-term infants > preterm infants.
Age of onset: much more frequent in the neonatal period than in other times of life.

H&E: **General:** may be symptomatic or asymptomatic depending on size and whether tension pneumothorax is present.
Asymptomatic: hyper-resonance and diminished breath sounds over the involved side of the chest.
Symptomatic: usually sudden deterioration with the following signs:
(1) **Asymmetry of the chest wall expansion.**
(2) **Respiratory distress:** tachypnoea, tachycardia, grunting, cyanosis.
(3) **Signs on the unaffected side:** intercostal/subcostal/sternal/substernal recession.
(4) **Signs on the affected side:** ↓breath sounds, hyper-resonant percussion.
(5) **Tension pneumothorax:** trachea and cardiac apex are deviated away from the affected side (late signs).
(6) **Shock:** may occur in tension pneumothorax due to compression of the great vessels and ↓cardiac output.

P: **Pathophysiology:** air from a ruptured alveolus escapes into the interstitial spaces of the lung, where it may cause interstitial emphysema or track down along the peribronchial and perivascular connective tissue sheaths to the base of the lung. With large volumes of escaped air there is subsequent formation of a pneumothorax, pneumomediastinum, or SC emphysema. Overdistension of alveoli is more likely to occur in immature lungs because of a decreased number of pores of Kohn which redistribute pressure between alveoli.

I: **CXR:** determine size of pneumothorax. In tension pneumothorax management should not be delayed by obtaining CXR.
ABG: may show respiratory compromise with hypoxia, hypercapnia +/− respiratory acidosis.

M: **Prevention:** infants requiring ventilatory support should be ventilated with the lowest pressures that provide adequate chest movement and satisfactory ABGs.
Emergency aspiration: in tension pneumothorax with a large bore cannula in the 2nd intercostal space midclavicular line.
Chest drain insertion: 4th–5th intercostal space midaxillary line; following emergency aspiration, in symptomatic pneumothorax or in infants with underlying respiratory disease.
Conservative management: in an asymptomatic infant without any underlying respiratory disease.

C: Usually no complications with adequate management.

P: Overall good prognosis. Can be fatal in neonates if not recognised promptly.

D: **Early onset of puberty:**
Females: development of 1° pubertal changes < 8 years or menarche < 10 years.
Males: development of 1° pubertal changes < 9 years.

A: **Central precocious puberty:** physiological normal pubertal development that is chronologically early. It results from hypothalamic GnRH-stimulated episodic gonadotrophin secretion (↑LH > FSH):

(1) **Idiopathic:** there is often no demonstrable underlying pathology (especially in females).
(2) **CNS dysfunction 2° to:**
- **Hypothalamic hamartoma:** most common type of CNS tumour that causes precocious puberty. It is a congenital malformation consisting of nerve tissue mass containing GnRH neurosecretory neurons.
- **Destruction from tumours:** craniopharyngioma, ganglioneuroma.
- **Destruction from space-occupying lesions:** arachnoid cysts.
- **Hydrocephalus.**
- **Infection:** brain abscess, encephalitis, meningitis.
- **Head trauma.**

Peripheral precocious puberty: pubertal development resulting from stimulation by a hormone other than hypothalamic GnRH, i.e. gonadotrophin-independent. May result from:

(1) **Inappropriate sex steroid synthesis 2° to:**
- Congenital adrenal hyperplasia.
- Tumours: adrenal, ovarian (granulosa cell), testicular (Leydig cell).
- McCune–Albright syndrome: characterised by hyperpigmented lesions similar to café-au-lait spots, polyostotic fibrous dysplasia and several endocrine disorders such as precocious puberty, toxic multinodular goitre, and amenorrhea-galactorrhea.

(2) **Exogenous sex steroids:** OCPs, topical oestrogens, and overuse of vaginal oestrogen (used in labial adhesions).

A/R: Family history (especially idiopathic central precocious puberty).

E: Rare disorder. Central is more common than peripheral. F > M.
Females are more likely to have idiopathic cause. Males are more likely to have organic cause.

H&E: **General:** early development of stages of puberty (Tanner stages; see Delayed puberty).
Specific: signs specific to individual syndromes, e.g. hyperpigmented lesions in McCune–Albright syndrome.

P: See **A**.

I: **Bloods:** LH/FSH/testosterone/oestrogen/LHRH levels.
Radiology:
(1) CT +/− MRI brain if neurological cause suspected.
(2) USS of the uterus and ovaries or testes.
(3) Wrist X-ray: for assessment of bone age.

M: A specialist paediatric endocrinologist should be involved. Organic causes should be investigated and managed appropriately. In idiopathic central precocious puberty, indications for treatment include the child's age of onset and rate of pubertal development.

C: May be associated with psychological problems. Other specific complications are associated with individual pathologies.

P: Mortality and morbidity ranges from mild to severe depending on aetiology; removal of exogenous sex steroids versus large unresectable cerebral tumours.

Precocious puberty (partial)

D: Early partial sexual development, characterised often by transient and minimal pubertal development in the absence of other stigmata of puberty. There are 3 categories:
Premature thelarche: isolated development of the breasts in infancy.
Premature adrenarche: pubic hair development before 8 years in females and 9 years in males.
Isolated premature menarche: premature vaginal bleeding.

A: **Premature thelarche:** due to period of relatively high but decreasing activity of the hypothalamic–pituitary–ovarian axis from age 6 months to 2 years.
Premature adrenarche: caused by early maturation of the normal pubertal adrenal androgen secretory mechanism.
Isolated premature menarche: spontaneous regression of an ovarian cyst, hypothyroidism, McCune–Albright syndrome; characterised by pigmented lesions similar to café-au-lait spots, polyostotic fibrous dysplasia, and several endocrine disorders including toxic multinodular goitre, amenorrhoea-galactorrhoea, and precocious puberty.

A/R: POS, obesity.

E: **Premature thelarche:** relatively common in girls <2 years of age.
Premature adrenarche: more common in Asian and African-Caribbean children.
Isolated premature menarche: uncommon.

H&E: **Premature thelarche:** unilateral or bilateral enlargement of the breasts may occur physiologically between the ages of 6 months and 2 years. It is non-progressive and not associated with areolar development.
Premature adrenarche: pubic hair development is usually self-limiting. It may be associated with a slight ↑ in growth rate.
Isolated premature menarche: may occur physiologically in the postnatal period. Must be distinguished from bloody foul-smelling discharge (trauma, foreign body, sexual abuse) and bleeding from the urinary tract. Obtain detailed history and examination to determine other causes (see **A**).

P: See **A**.

I: **General:** may not be necessary with premature thelarche.
Pathology: LH/FSH/oestrogen levels, GnRH testing, ACTH testing (defects in steroidogenesis).
Radiology: USS of ovaries and uterus, bone age radiography.
Culture: urine, vaginal discharge (premature menarche).

M: A specialist paediatric endocrinologist should be involved. Normally no intervention is required and management consists of investigation to exclude evidence of complete precocious puberty and regular follow-up.

C: **Premature thelarche:** can progress to precocious puberty.
Premature adrenarche: may progress to POS, or develop clinical features and hormonal evidence of excessive androgen synthesis in adolescence.
Isolated premature menarche: usually no complications.
Psychosocial impact: difficulties associated with not developing at the same speed as peers.

P: Usually good. Most children go on to have normal puberty and no deficit in final adult stature.

D: A chronic inflammatory skin disease characterised by well-demarcated erythematous plaques covered by silvery scales.

A: **Genetic factors:** studies have shown 30–60% of affected children have a 1st degree relative with psoriasis.
Environmental factors (precipitants/exacerbants): psycho-emotional stress (80%), viral and bacterial infections (50%), e.g. streptococcal infection, winter, sunlight, trauma, medications (β-blockers, antimalarials).

A/R: **HLA types:** CW6, B13, and B17.

E: **Incidence:** 1–3% of the world's population.
Age of onset: <2 years: 2%, <5 years: 6.5%, <10 years: 10%, <15 years: 27%, <20 years: 37%.
Race: commoner in Caucasians. F : M = 2 : 1 (Norwegian psoriasis study).

H: **Infants:** intractable nappy rash.
Children: itching or occasionally tender skin.
Auspitz phenomenon: pinpoint bleeding with removal of scales.
Koebner phenomenon: skin lesions develop at the site of trauma/scars.

E: Well-demarcated, erythematous, scaling papules and plaques. Children commonly have facial lesions. Nail pitting and onycholysis is rare in children.
Guttate psoriasis: commonest presentation in children 5–12 years old; small, drop-like plaques over trunk, limbs; occurs post streptococcal infection (tonsillitis), usually resolves over 3–4 months.
Plaque psoriasis: less common; well-defined, disc-shaped plaques on elbows, knees, scalp hair margin, or sacrum, covered by silvery scales.
Napkin psoriasis: well-defined eruption in nappy area of infants.
Generalised pustular psoriasis (rare): acute development of sheets of yellow pustules on erythematous background with associated fever.

P: Rapid epidermal proliferation (20× normal), possibly driven by cytokines released by T lymphocytes in the dermis, and associated accelerated upward migration of immature keratinocytes.

I: Majority do not need investigating as psoriasis is a clinical diagnosis.
Guttate psoriasis: ASOT, throat swab.
Nail involvement: analyse nail clippings to exclude fungal infection.

M: **Topical:** emollients for moisturisation, coal tar (↓DNA synthesis), dithranol (anti-mitotic, irritates normal skin, stains), topical steroids (moderately potent, e.g. eumovate), vitamin D_3 analogue (e.g. calcipotriol, inhibits cell proliferation and stimulates keratinocyte differentiation).
UV Light: oral PUVA or UVB (for widespread thin lesions or guttate psoriasis).
Systemic: in severe cases use methotrexate (anti-inflammatory and immune modulatory, risk of liver cirrhosis, teratogenic), cyclosporin (immunosuppressant), retinoids (for pustular psoriasis), etanercept (anti-TNFα; especially for psoriatic arthritis).
Advice: avoid exacerbating factors.

C: **Seronegative arthritides:**
(1) Distal asymmetrical oligoarthritis (DIP joints).
(2) Dactylitis (IP arthritis and flexor tenosynovitis).
(3) Rheumatoid arthritis–like (symmetrical polyarthritis).
(4) Arthritis mutilans (telescoping of the digits).
(5) Ankylosing spondylitis.
Other complications: anterior uveitis, erythroderma.

P: Chronic/relapsing disease. Generalised pustular psoriasis is life-threatening.

Pulmonary stenosis

D: Acyanotic obstructive heart disease; may be valvular, subvalvular (infundibular), or supravalvular. These lesions are associated collectively with obstruction to right ventricular outflow; mild <30 mmHg, moderate 30–50 mmHg, severe >50 mmHg.

A: The development of pulmonary valvular stenosis is due to abnormal development of the pulmonary valve tissue and distal portion of the bulbous cordis.

A/R: Other congenital heart defects; ASD, VSD, PDA.

E: Represents 8–12% of all congenital heart defects. Occurs in as many as 50% of all patients with other congenital cardiac lesions. M = F.

H: **Mild stenosis:** most children are asymptomatic in infancy and childhood.
Moderate stenosis: dyspnoea and fatigue appear as severity and decompensation increases.
Severe stenosis: may present with exercise intolerance, angina on exertion, and heart failure. Rarely, severe stenosis may present with cyanosis due to right → left shunting through the foramen ovale or an associated ASD.

E: **Mild to moderate stenosis:** child is usually acyanotic with a right ventricular heave +/− systolic thrill, S1 is followed by a click and S2 is delayed, systolic murmur is heard loudest at the left upper sternal border, radiating to the back; the severity of stenosis is directly related to intensity and duration of the murmur.
Severe stenosis: cyanosis, signs of heart failure with tricuspid insufficiency; giant 'a' waves in JVP, hepatomegaly, and a pulsatile liver.

P: Fusion of the leaflet commissures results in a thickened and domed appearance to the valve.

I: **CXR:** normal heart size, post-stenotic dilatation of PA, ↓pulmonary blood flow. May show signs of CHF with right ventricular and atrial enlargement.
ECG: normal in mild stenosis, but in severe stenosis may show right axis deviation, RVH, and signs of right heart strain.
Doppler echo: diagnostic and determines severity of stenosis.

M: **Valvular pulmonary stenosis:** management determined by the Doppler gradient:
(1) **Mild:** no treatment, follow-up screening examination and ECG for 3–5 years.
(2) **Moderate:** depends on whether symptomatic, and weighing up of risk/benefit ratio.
(3) **Severe:** proceed to cardiac catheterisation +/− balloon valvuloplasty or valvotomy.
Infundibular and supravalvular pulmonary stenosis: if severe, require operative and invasive surgical intervention.

C: RVH and CHF in severe pulmonary stenosis.

P: Mild valvular pulmonary stenosis usually does not progress, but the moderate to severe disease does.
Following balloon or surgical valvotomy, the prognosis is excellent. RVH regresses and the condition does not recur. Life expectancy is similar to the general population and most patients remain asymptomatic.

Pyloric stenosis

D: Anatomical and functional obstruction of the GI tract due to localised hypertrophy and hyperplasia of the pylorus muscle.

A: **Genetic component:** identical twin studies have shown 80–90% concordance.
There is speculation on the role of gastrin and myenteric plexus abnormalities.

A/R: **Family history:** 5–10% of infants have previously affected parents, first-born children.

E: 1/200 live births; the most common cause of intestinal obstruction in infancy, commoner in Caucasians.
Sex: M : F = 1 : 4

H: Usually presents at 2–6 weeks but may present up to 6 months of age.
Characteristic history:
(1) Progressive non-bilious vomiting within 30 min of a feed, which may become projectile. May occasionally be associated with coffee-ground vomiting 2° to gastritis or Mallory–Weiss tear at the gastroesophageal junction.
(2) Persistently hungry following projectile vomiting.
(3) Constipation.
(4) Failure to thrive.

E: **Systemic:** weight loss +/− signs of dehydration, ↓skin turgor, sunken fontanelle, ↓urinary output, may be jaundiced (5%).
GI: visible peristalsis from left to right in the left upper quadrant during a feed. An olive-sized pyloric mass may be palpated in the right upper quadrant during a feed or immediately after a vomit.

P: Marked hypertrophy and hyperplasia of the 2 (circular and longitudinal) muscular layers of the pylorus occurs, which → narrowing of the gastric antrum. The pyloric canal becomes lengthened and the whole pylorus becomes thickened. The mucosa is usually oedematous and thickened. In advanced cases, the stomach is markedly dilated.

I: **Bloods:** U&E for hypochloraemic hypokalaemic alkalosis due to vomiting; ↑pH, ↓K^+, ↓Cl^-, ↓Na^{2+}, ↑HCO_3^-, ↑urea. May have mild, unconjugated hyperbilirubinaemia.
USS abdomen: performed in most cases where pyloric stenosis is suspected.

M: **Pre-op:** fluid resuscitation and correction of electrolyte imbalance. NG tube is required to relieve gastric contents.
Ramstedt pyloromyotomy: an incision is made in the pyloric canal to divide the hypertrophied muscle fibres down to, but not through, the pyloric mucosa.

C: Surgical intervention prevents complications without which dehydration and electrolyte disturbance are usually fatal.

P: Excellent following surgery. Surgery carries < 1% mortality rate. Feeding is introduced gradually post-operatively.

Recurrent abdominal pain

D: Abdominal pain sufficient to interrupt normal activities.

A: **Functional abdominal pain:** 90% of children who experience recurrent abdominal pain have no structural or mucosal abnormality in the GI tract.
Specific GI disorders: 10% of recurrent abdominal pain is due to IBS, non-ulcer dyspepsia, and abdominal migraine.

A/R: Stress at home/school, anxiety.

E: **Incidence:** 10% of school-age children.

H: **Functional abdominal pain:** pain is characteristically around the umbilicus, does not wake the child at night, and is not associated with food, feeding, or bowel habit. The child is otherwise well.
IBS: pain is often worse before and relieved by defaecation, stools have excess mucous; children experience bloating, sensation of incomplete defaecation, and constipation.
Non-ulcer dyspepsia: epigastric pain, post-prandial vomiting, early satiety, and acid reflux.
Abdominal migraine: pain is paroxysmal, stereotypic, and may be associated with facial pallor +/− headache (throbbing, unilateral, aura).

E: There may be no findings or mild generalised abdominal tenderness.

P: **IBS:** abnormal contractions of the intestines, which are modulated by fluctuating levels of stress and anxiety.
Non-ulcer dyspepsia: abnormal gastric motility.
Abdominal migraine: classical cranial migraine is associated with abdominal pain, in children the abdominal pain can predominate.

I: **Investigations should only be performed if clinically indicated.**
Urine analysis and culture may be performed to exclude a UTI.

M: **Education:** the diagnosis of functional abdominal pain should be made as a positive diagnosis rather than a diagnosis of exclusion, or the child will be exposed to unnecessary investigations.
Medical: famotidine (H_2-blocker), pizotifen (antihistamine and serotonin antagonist), and peppermint oil enteric-coated capsules have been shown to ↓ measured pain outcomes of recurrent abdominal pain when compared with others in control groups. There was greater improvement when therapy was targeted to the specific GI disorder (dyspepsia, abdominal migraine, IBS). Using drugs can, however, risk somatising a functional, usually self-limiting, disorder.
Behavioural: CBT and biofeedback have been shown to be effective in decreasing pain scores. The behavioural interventions seem to have a general positive effect on children with true functional abdominal pain.
Dietary: studies that have evaluated dietary interventions have had conflicting results in the case of fibre, or showed no efficacy in the case of lactose avoidance.

C: Functional abdominal pain may become a strategy of school avoidance. If not tackled effectively, this may affect the child's school performance, and → further behavioural problems.

P: 50% of children affected with functional abdominal pain resolve rapidly. In 25% the pain resolves in a few months, and in 25% the symptoms continue into adulthood as IBS.

D: A significant deterioration in renal function occurring over hours or days, resulting in ↑plasma urea, creatinine, and oliguria. Complete recovery of renal function usually occurs within days/weeks.

A: **Pre-renal:**
(1) Hypovolaemia (haemorrhage, GI losses, DKA, burns, diarrhoea, septic shock).
(2) Cardiac failure (severe coarctation, hypoplastic left heart, myocarditis).
(3) Hypoxia (pneumonia, RDS).

Intrinsic renal:
(1) ATN (80% of causes) due to circulatory compromise or nephrotoxic drugs (paracetamol, aminoglycosides).
(2) Acute GN (see chapter).
(3) Acute interstitial nephritis (infection, drugs; NSAIDs, frusemide, penicillin).
(4) Small/large vessel obstruction (renal artery/vein thrombosis, vasculitis, HUS, TTP).

Post-renal (obstructive):
(1) Neuropathic bladder; may be acute in transverse myelitis, spinal trauma.
(2) Stones (bilateral pelviureteric junction or ureteral)
(3) Urethral prolapse of bladder ureterocele.

A/R: Acute illnesses and multiorgan failure.

E: 0.8/100 000 children.

H: Vomiting, anorexia, oliguria, convulsions, previous sore throat and fever (post-streptococcal GN), bloody diarrhoea and progressive pallor (HUS), drug history.

E: Assess intravascular volume status: volume depleted (cool peripheries, tachycardia, postural hypotension) or overloaded. Is patient septic? Is patient obstructed? Examine abdomen for palpable bladder.

P: **Acute tubular necrosis:**
Macro: enlarged kidneys with pale cortex. **Micro:** swelling and necrosis of the tubular cells, interstitial oedema with macrophage and plasma cell infiltration.

I: **Bloods:** ↓Hb (hypovolaemia/haemorrhage), ↑WCC, ↑CRP, blood cultures (sepsis), ↑urea, ↑creatinine, ↑K^+, ↑phosphate, ↓Ca^{2+}, ↓ Mg^{2+}, LFTs, venous capillary blood gas, clotting (DIC), ASOT (post-streptococcal GN).
Blood film: HUS/TTP (RBC fragmentation).
Urine: Urinalysis for blood, protein (GN), glucose (interstitial nephritis), microscopy for casts (GN), urine Na^+, urea, creatinine, osmolality to differentiate between pre-renal and intrinsic renal failure.
ECG: signs of hyperkalaemia; tall tented T waves → small or absent P waves →↑P–R interval → widened QRS complex → sine wave pattern → asystole.
CXR: signs of pulmonary oedema.
Renal USS: in ARF, kidneys appear normal or increased in size and echogenicity, may detect stones or clot in RVT.
Renal biopsy: if diagnosis has not been determined.

M: **Resuscitate:** especially in pre-renal causes of ATN.
Monitor: daily U&E, temperature, PR, RR, BP, O_2 saturation, hourly urine output, CVP, daily weights.
Treat cause: avoid potential causative drugs, post-renal causes; catheters, stents, nephrostomy or surgery, hypovolaemia; fluids, sepsis; antibiotics.
Nutrition: high-calorie intake, with enteral/parenteral nutrition if oral intake is poor.

Dialysis: indications for acute dialysis:

(1) Severe extracellular fluid volume overload; ↑BP, pulmonary oedema not responding to diuretics.
(2) Severe $\uparrow K^+$; not responding to medical treatment.
(3) Severe systematic uraemia.
(4) Severe metabolic acidosis, not controllable with IV sodium bicarbonate.
(5) Removal of toxins (drugs, poisons).

C: Heart failure and pulmonary oedema (volume overload), GI bleeding (gastric ulceration, gastritis, and platelet dysfunction), muscle wasting due to hypercatabolic state, uraemic pericarditis/encephalopathy.

P: Depends on the causative factor. Recovery of renal function following ARF is most likely following pre-renal causes, HUS, ATN, acute interstitial nephritis, or uric acid nephropathy.

D: Characterised by ↓GFR, persistently ↑urea and ↑creatinine concentration.

A: **Age < 5 years:** congenital abnormalities (hypoplasia, dysplasia, obstruction (posterior urethral valve), malformations).
Age > 5 years:
(1) Hereditary disorders: Alport syndrome (thickened glomerular basement membrane), infantile polycystic disease.
(2) All causes of GN and tubulo-interstitial nephritis may → CRF (see GN chapter).
(3) VUR.
(4) Systemic disease (HSP, SLE).

A/R: See **A**.

E: Rare in children.

H: **Clinical presentations:** antenatal diagnosis, failure to thrive, delayed puberty, malaise, anorexia, anaemia, incidental (blood test/urinalysis).

E: Examine flanks for palpable kidneys (polycystic disease), pallor, oedema, pigmentation, scratch marks, hypertension, growth retardation, and rickets.

P: Progressive fibrosis of the glomeruli, tubules, and small vessels → renal scarring.

I: **Bloods:** ↓Hb, MCV (usually normocytic) $\downarrow Na^+$, $\uparrow K^+$, ↑urea, ↑creatinine, $\downarrow Ca^{2+}$, ↑phosphate, ↑ALP, ↑PTH (2° hyperparathyroidism).
Urine: 24-h collection for protein and creatinine clearance.
X-rays: for signs of osteomalacia and hyperparathyroidism.
Renal USS: for anatomical/hereditary abnormalities, measure size (small shrunken kidneys consistent with CRF), exclude obstruction/stones.
Renal biopsy: for changes specific to the underlying disease, contraindicated in shrunken kidneys.

M: **Monitor:** child's clinical (physical examination, growth, BP) and biochemical status.
Factors to treat:
(1) **A**naemia.
(2) **B**P control.
(3) **C**a^{2+} maintenance: 1-hydroxylated vitamin D analogues, e.g. alfacalcidol.
(4) **D**iet: high-energy intake, restrict K^+ in hyperkalaemia or acidosis, restriction of phosphate intake combined with use of phosphate binders to prevent 2° hyperparathyroidism.
(5) **D**rugs: avoid nephrotoxic drugs, adjust doses of other drugs, e.g. frusemide in oedema.
Continuous ambulatory peritoneal dialysis: dialysate is introduced and exchanged through a catheter, inserted via an SC tunnel into the peritoneum. Preferred method in children.
Haemodialysis: blood is removed via an arteriovenous fistula surgically constructed in the forearm to provide high flow. Uraemic toxins are removed by diffusion across a semipermeable membrane in an extracorporeal circuit.
Transplantation: in end-stage renal failure. Requires long-term immunosuppressants to ↓ rejection.

C: **Haematological:** anaemia, abnormal platelet activity (bruising, epistaxis).
Cardiovascular: accelerated atherosclerosis, ↑BP, and pericarditis.
Neurological: peripheral and autonomic neuropathy, proximal myopathy.
Renal osteodystrophy: osteoporosis, osteomalacia, 2°/3° hyperparathyroidism.
Endocrine: amenorrhoea.
Peritoneal dialysis: peritonitis (e.g. *Staphylococcus epidermidis*).

Haemodialysis:

(1) Acute: hypotension due to excessive removal of extracellular fluid.
(2) Long-term: atherosclerosis, sepsis (2° peritonitis with *Staph. aureus* infection).
(3) Amyloidosis: → periarticular deposition, arthralgia (e.g. shoulder) and carpal tunnel syndrome.

Transplantation/immunosuppression: opportunistic infections (e.g. *Pneumocystis carinii*), malignancies (lymphomas and skin), and side-effects of immunosuppressant drugs.

P: Depends on complications. Timely dialysis/transplantation improves survival.

D: Respiratory compromise in the newborn preterm infant 2° to surfactant deficiency.

A: The clinical syndrome of RDS arises from the interplay of a number of factors:
- Small lung volumes due to immaturity.
- Surfactant deficiency that → high alveolar surface tension, alveolar collapse, and intrapleural right → left shunting.
- **1° surfactant deficiency:** due to prematurity and promoted by hypoxia, acidosis, hypothermia, and hypotension during the delivery.
- **2° surfactant deficiency:** intrapartum asphyxia, pulmonary infections or haemorrhage, meconium aspiration, pneumonia.
- Soft thoracic cage means that as the neonate attempts to generate a large negative intrathoracic pressure the ribs and sternum 'cave in' and the abdominal contents are displaced downwards. This type of breathing is ineffective and → classical 'see-saw' breathing.

A/R: Preterm delivery, maternal DM, Caesarean section delivery infants, second-born twins, family history.

E: 50% of infants born at 28–32 weeks gestation develop RDS. The majority of infants < 28 weeks have RDS.

H&E: **Progressive signs of respiratory distress:** tachypnoea, grunting (expiration against partially closed glottis), subcostal and intercostal recession, nasal flaring, and with extremely premature infants apnoea +/− hypothermia may develop, and cyanosis.

P: **Macroscopic:** lungs appear airless and ruddy (liver-like).
Microscopic: diffuse atelectasis of the distal airspaces with distension of some of the distal airways and perilymphatic areas.

I: **ABG:**
(1) Respiratory acidosis due to alveolar atelectasis +/− overdistension of terminal airways.
(2) Metabolic acidosis due to lactic acidosis 2° to poor tissue perfusion.
(3) Hypoxia due to right → left shunting.
CXR: bilateral diffuse reticular granular or ground glass appearance, air bronchograms, and poor lung expansion.
Echo: to determine presence of PDA.

M: **Prevention:**
- Identification of at-risk infants, neonatologist/NICU early involvement.
- Amniocentesis for estimation of foetal lung maturity by lecithin/sphingomyelin ratio and presence of phosphatidylglycerol in at-risk infants.
- The prudent use of antenatal steroids stimulates foetal surfactant production and is used when preterm delivery is anticipated.

Treatment:
- Surfactant replacement therapy; reduces mortality from RDS by 40%.
- Correction of hypoglycaemia, hypothermia, and electrolyte imbalances.
- Oxygen and CPAP via nasal cannulae, ventilation either conventional or oscillatory.
- Prophylactic antibiotics to prevent respiratory infections.

C: **Acute:** alveolar rupture → pneumothorax, intracranial haemorrhage, periventricular leucomalacia (ischaemic necrosis of periventricular white matter), PDA, pulmonary haemorrhage, NEC, or GI perforation.
Chronic: CLD of prematurity, ROP, neurological impairment.

P: Previously extremely poor (60% mortality) but improving with antenatal steroids, surfactant therapy, and better techniques in ventilation.

Retinopathy of prematurity (ROP)

D: Serious vasoproliferative disorder affecting extremely preterm infants.

A: Infants at highest risk for ROP are those with the lowest birth weight and gestational age although many other factors are associated with ↑risk:
(1) Severity of general illness.
(2) Prolonged exposure to high concentrations of supplemental oxygen.
(3) Persistent acidosis, period of mechanical ventilation.
(4) Presence of a PDA.
(5) IVH.

A/R: See **A**.

E: Incidence varies with birth weight, 50–70% of infants whose weight is less than 1250 g at birth have some degree of ROP. African-Caribbean patients appear to have less severe disease. M = F.

H: All neonates who are at risk should be screened: gestational age < 32 weeks, birth weight < 1500 g. Screening begins at 4 weeks of age and continues until the retina is seen to be fully vascularised.

E: Should be performed by an experienced ophthalmologist. International classification system for ROP uses disease zones 1–3 which measures extent of retina involved, stage of disease, which measures severity and 'plus' disease (tortuous dilated retinal vessels) which implies active progressive disease.

P: The retinal vasculature begins to form in the 16th week of gestation. Retinal vessels grow out of the optic disc as a wave of mesenchymal spindle cells. In preterm infants normal retinal vascular maturation is interrupted. The blood vessels constrict and atrophy, which disrupts the blood supply to the retina and causes ischaemia. Angiogenic factors (e.g. vascular endothelial growth factor) are released from the mesenchymal spindle cells and the ischaemic retina and → new vessel proliferation. New vessels are tortuous and fragile and may haemorrhage, which results in fibrosis and subsequently retinal detachment.

I: Diagnosis is based on findings of clinical examination.

M: **Prevention:** likelihood is reduced with careful control of pO_2 in the ventilated child and use of O_2 concentrations of < 40%.
Neonatal screening: studies have shown that ablative therapy to destroy the avascular areas of the retina in threshold disease improves outcome.
Ablative surgery:
Cryotherapy (freezing): requires general or local anaesthesia.
Complications: intraocular haemorrhage, conjunctival haematoma or laceration, and bradycardia.
Laser therapy: preferred option to cryotherapy as the ocular tissues are less traumatised, general anaesthesia is avoided, and there are fewer complications. Complications: cataracts, intraocular haemorrhages.

C: Severe visual impairment, myopia, amblyopia, and strabismus.

P: Patients should receive yearly ophthalmology follow-up as the long-term visual sequelae need early detection and intervention.

D: A systemic inflammatory disorder affecting the heart, joints, CNS, skin, and SC tissue, characterised by an exudative and proliferative inflammatory lesion of the connective tissue.

A: Follows 0.3% of group A β-streptococcal infection usually of the URT.

A/R: Malnutrition, overcrowding, socio-economically disadvantaged groups.

E: Still common in developing countries; however, has decreased in developed countries due to ↑use of penicillin. **Peak age:** 5–15 years. M = F.

H&E: Rheumatic fever occurs ~20 days after streptococcal throat infection.
Diagnosed by modified Duckett Jones criteria (2 major or 1 major and 2 minor):

Major:
(1) Carditis
(2) Migratory polyarthritis
(3) Erythema marginatum (serpiginous flat, nonscarring painless rash)
(4) SC nodules
(5) Sydenham's chorea (rapid uncoordinated jerky movements primarily of hands, feet and face)

Minor:
(1) Fever
(2) Arthralgia
(3) Previous rheumatic fever or carditis
(4) Positive ESR/CRP
(5) Leucocytosis
(6) Prolonged PR interval

Presentation can be of sudden onset, typically beginning with a polyarthritis 2–6 weeks after streptococcal pharyngitis, and is usually characterised by pyrexia and toxicity.
Presentation may be of insidious onset with mild carditis, usually as a result of a sub-clinical infection.

P: **Joints:** non-specific oedema and hyperaemia of inflamed synovial membranes.
Cardiac: acute interstitial valvulitis causing valvular oedema, thickening, fusion, and retraction of leaflets and cusps. This results in valvular stenosis or regurgitation. Aschoff bodies are found in the myocardium.
Skin: nodule biopsies resemble Aschoff bodies.

I: No investigation is pathognomonic; diagnosis is confirmed using the modified Duckett Jones criteria.
Bloods: ↑ESR/CRP, ↑WCC, ASOT. **Throat swab:** MC+S.
Local inflammation: ↑WCC with negative cultures in synovial fluid (usually clear/yellow).
ECG: PR prolongation in acute carditis.
ECHO: mitral regurgitation, myocarditis, pericarditis.

M: **Treat infection:** IV pencillin or cephalosporins.
Arthritis: analgesics such as codeine or NSAIDs in mild cases, aggressive use of anti-inflammatory drugs may be required in severe cases.
Carditis: NSAIDs to suppress inflammation. In severe carditis with heart failure corticosteroids (prednisolone) may be started.
Antistreptococcal prophylaxis: penicillin V orally for 25 years to prevent recurrence.

C: Repeated streptococcal infections, damage to the heart valves (especially mitral and aortic stenosis), endocarditis, heart failure, arrhythmias, and pericarditis.

P: **Duration of illness:** in 75% of cases the acute attack lasts 6 weeks, 90% have resolved in 12 weeks, and only 5% of patients have symptoms that persist for $>$6 months.

Risk factors for CRHD: include the severity of the initial carditis, the presence or absence of recurrences, and the amount of time since the episode of rheumatic fever.

Incidence of CRHD: at 10 years after initial presentation, incidence of CRHD is 34% in patients without recurrences but 60% in patients with recurrent rheumatic fever.

Scabies

D: Eruptive skin reaction caused by mite infestation.

A: **Infestation by arthropod *Sarcoptes scabiei*:** The adult female mite is 0.3–0.5 mm long and has 4 pairs of legs. The average patient is infected with 10–15 live adult female mites at any given time.
Mechanism of spread: via prolonged direct human contact (> 20 min) such as holding hands or playing contact games. Scabies is often incorrectly viewed as an STD since one common means of transmission is by being in the same bed with an infected person. Fomite transmission is possible from towels, bedding, underclothing, and even toilet seats.

A/R: Not always a disease of overcrowding or poor living conditions.

E: May be observed in people of all ages.

H: **Itch:** occurs 2–6 weeks after infestation, worse at night and in warm conditions; may remain for many weeks after the mites are killed as irritants remain in the skin until that part of the skin is shed.
In young infants: irritability, especially during sleep may be the only symptom.

E: **Burrows:** tortuous erythematous tracts with the mite (occasionally visible) in a vesicle at one end; are pathognomonic but hard to identify in the presence of 2° infection due to excoriations, papules, vesicles, and pustules.
Rash: itchy, ill-defined urticarial hypersensitivity reaction 2–6 weeks after infestation due to sensitivity to mite eggs and faeces. May be confused with eczema.
Distribution:
Neonates: head, neck, and face can be involved.
Infants and younger children: palms, soles, and trunk.
Older children: webs between fingers and toes, axillae, wrists (flexor aspects), abdomen (waistband area), around nipples, penis, and buttocks.

P: Lesions are caused by the gravid female mite burrowing beneath the stratum corneum. She leaves behind a trail of debris, eggs, and faeces, which induces a hypersensitivity response.

I: **Scabies is mainly a clinical diagnosis:**
Mites, eggs, and faeces may be seen in skin scrapings from lesions under microscopic examination.

M: **Treat child and all close/family contacts.**
(1) Malathion/permethrin lotion is the treatment of choice; apply to all areas below the neck overnight. Resistance to these treatments is becoming more common.
(2) Benzyl benzoate emulsion may be applied; however, it smells bad and is an irritant.
(3) Mittens in children < 2 years to prevent excoriation and 2° infection.
(4) Rash and itch take a few weeks to settle, treat with topical steroids.
(5) Wash towels and linen in hot water.

C: **2° bacterial infection:** impetigo requires treatment with topical mupirocin.
Psychosocial impact: 2° to stigma associated with infestation.

P: Good with appropriate treatment, environmental eradication, and treatment of contacts.

D: Significant child-motivated refusal to attend school and/or difficulties remaining in class for a whole day.

A: **Separation anxiety disorder:** separation anxiety is part of normal development until the age of 3–4 years after which it may have adverse effects on development and social interactions and may → school refusal and other behavioural problems.

Environmental: distress associated with an issue related to school attendance: peer group interactions; bullying (physical, psychological) and academic performance–related (examinations, presentations).

A/R: **Parental separation anxiety disorder:** associated with overprotective, needy, or depressed parent. **Adverse life events:** death in family, divorce.

E: Peaks at the age of entry into new schools, e.g. 5 years and 11 years as well as during adolescence 14–15 years. Overall prevalence rate ~2–5%. Slightly more prevalent in lower socio-economic group families.

H&E: Use structured diagnostic interview to elicit the reasons behind refusal.

Range of presentation: entirely absent from school, leaving before end of school day, crying, clinging, tantrums, or other intense behaviour prior to going to school, exhibiting unusual distress during school days that → pleas for future absenteeism.

Can be grouped into 2 types of problematic behaviour:

(1) **Internalisation:** generalised worrying, fatigue, physical complaints (stomach aches, nausea, and headaches), social anxiety and isolation.

(2) **Externalisation:** tantrums, aggressive behaviour (verbal and physical).

Screen for depression: low mood, anhedonia, feelings of worthlessness.

Screen for other behavioural problems: sleep disorders, eating disorders, conduct disorders, drug abuse.

Screen for symptoms and signs of organic cause: lethargy, failure to thrive, pallor, psychomotor retardation, polyuria and polydipsia, focal neurological signs.

P: **Reinforcement of behaviour patterns:**

Negative reinforcement: tantrums allow children to avoid distressing situations.

Positive reinforcement: obtaining more enjoyment, e.g. playing computer games at home instead of working at school.

I: No investigations are done by most community paediatricians.

If organic cause suspected: FBC, TFTs, urine dipstick for glycosuria.

Urine toxicology (if indicated): for drugs of abuse.

MRI/CT: if suggestive of neurological cause.

M: Early stepwise return to school, which is tolerable to the child. Close liaison with the school.

CBT: encourages more assertive and adapting approaches to school attendance, toleration of separation; using modelling, role-playing, and relaxation techniques.

Medical: SSRIs (e.g. fluoxetine) may be appropriate in certain children who show signs of depression.

C: Deteriorating school performance, social isolation, family tension/conflict, reduced probability of attending higher education. Substance abuse, anxiety, and depression in adulthood.

P: Related to duration of refusal before treatment onset. Complications are more likely to develop the longer the delay in dealing with the problem.

Septicaemia

D: **Bacteraemia:** proliferation of bacteria in the circulation.
Septicaemia: systemic response to infection; tachypnoea, tachycardia, and fever or hypothermia.
Sepsis syndrome/SIRS: evidence of reduced end-organ perfusion (oliguria/altered GCS) with elevated lactate levels.
Septic shock: sepsis syndrome plus hypotension that does not respond to fluid therapy.

A: **Early onset neonatal sepsis:** usually multiorgan system disease with respiratory failure, meningitis, circulatory shock, and ATN due to GBS or *E. coli*.
Late onset neonatal sepsis: usually occurs in full-term infant due to *Neisseria meningitidis*, *Streptococcus pneumoniae*, Hib, HSV, CMV or enteroviruses.
Hospital-acquired: occurs predominantly among preterm infants in NICU due to *Staphylococcus aureus*, *Staph. epidermidis* or gram-negative organisms.
Immunocompromised septicaemia: infected by broader spectrum of pathogens including fungi.
Older children: usually caused by *Neisseria meningitides* or *Strep. pneumoniae*.

A/R: **Neonatal early onset:** vaginal colonisation with GBS, PROM (>24 h term, >18 h preterm infants), preterm delivery.
Medical instrumentation: indwelling central venous lines and ET tubes, peritoneal dialysis, surgery, and prosthetic heart valves.

E: Commonest cause of bacteraemia is pneumococcus. Commonest cause of septic shock is meningococcal septicaemia.

H&E: **Determine immunisation status.**
Presentation depends on the 1° system affected:
CNS: bulging fontanelle (neonates), headache, photophobia, neck stiffness, seizures, ↓GCS.
Respiratory: tachypneoa, apnoea, grunting, cyanosis.
Cardiovascular: tachycardia, hypotension.
GI: poor feeding, abdominal pain, vomiting, diarrhoea.
General: lethargy, fever, hypothermia, purpuric rash.

P: **Septic shock results from the following components:**
(1) Gram-positive bacteria peptidoglycans.
(2) Gram-negative bacteria lipopolysaccharides.
(3) Host response: release of inflammatory cytokines, coagulation cascade, prostaglandins and NO → vasodilatation, ↑capillary permeability and shift in intravascular compartment; resulting in hypotension.

TSS: *Staph. aureus* and *Strep. pyogenes* may act as 'superantigens' that activate entire classes of T cells and initiate a particularly severe form of SIRS.

I: **Bloods:** ↑/↓WCC (neutropaenia/neutrophilia), ↑CRP, U&E, blood glucose, clotting, ABG (hypoxia, metabolic acidosis).
Radiology: CXR, USS abdomen if intra-abdominal sepsis is suspected.
Microscopy, culture and sensitivity: MSU, blood (×3 different sites), CSF (LP if vital signs are stable enough to tolerate procedure).

M: **Transfer to NICU/PICU:**
Supportive: fluid resuscitation +/− inotropes to maintain BP and perfusion, adequate oxygenation by non-invasive or ventilatory means.
Empirical antimicrobial therapy: neonatal septicaemia; ceftriaxone and ampicillin. Vancomycin and gentamicin in hospital-acquired infections, wider spectrum cover for immunocompromised patients.
Prevention: immunisation (+ pneumococcus in at-risk infants). Intrapartum penicillin in mothers colonised with GBS or PROM, previous GBS infant.

C: Multiorgan failure, DIC, residual neurological deficit.

P: **Mortality:** septic shock 40–70%; multiorgan failure 90–100%.

D: A child's height that is below the 2nd centile for gender and sex.

A: **Familial:** many short children have a normal centile target range when compared to midparental height and not the normal population. These children have bone age appropriate for chronological age and a normal growth velocity. Care must be taken to exclude an inherited growth disorder affecting parents and child.

IUGR: 33% of infants with severe IUGR remain short as do extremely preterm infants.

Constitutional delay of growth and puberty (see Delayed puberty): may be induced by dieting or excessive exercise.

Endocrine: children usually short and overweight. Caused by hypothyroidism; congenital or autoimmune thyroiditis in adolescence, GH deficiency (may be due to craniopharyngioma which affects the pituitary), corticosteroid excess (usually iatrogenic). The hallmark of endocrine disease is ↓ in linear growth occurring to a greater degree than weight loss and delay of bone age.

Nutritional/chronic illness: relatively common cause with children being short and underweight; caused by malnutrition from insufficient food intake, unbalanced diets, or anorexia associated with an underlying chronic disease (coeliac disease, CD, CRF, CF, CHF, and chronic hypoxia).

Psychological: emotional deprivation/neglect.

Chromosomal disorders: Down syndrome, Turner syndrome (45XO), Silver–Russell syndrome, Noonan syndrome, Prader–Willi syndrome.

Disproportion: short-limbed dysplasia, achondroplasia, mucopolysaccharidoses.

A/R: See **A**.

E: By definition 2% of the paediatric population has short stature; there are normal variations related to ethnic background.

H: **General:**

(1) Original birth records should be obtained to confirm length, weight, and frontal occipital circumference.

(2) Parent's height and weight should be determined and pubertal timing in 1st degree relatives.

(3) Boys: target height (cm) $= \frac{FH + MH}{2} + 7$.

(4) Girls: target height (cm) $= \frac{FH + MH}{2} - 7$.

Specific:

(1) Review of symptoms by organ system as this may indicate an underlying disease.

(2) Detailed social history should also be obtained; sports history, refugee status, and home situation.

E: **Measure:** height (measured whilst standing in triplicate using a calibrated wall-mounted stadiometer), weight, and frontal–occipital circumference in infants.

Long bone growth: in children who cannot stand or recline completely (spina bifida, contractures), arm span provides a reliable alternative for longitudinal assessment of long bone growth.

Growth velocity: can be calculated as the change in standing height over at least 6/12 for children or change in length over 4/12 for infants.

Specific: height of sitting body (short-limbed dwarfism), thyroid examination, ulcerative stomatitis (CD), midfacial hypoplasia (GH deficiency), neck-webbing, widely spaced nipples (Turner syndrome), frontal bossing, short limbs (achondroplasia), cushingoid face, central obesity, ↑BP (Cushing syndrome).

P: See **A**.

I: **Bloods:** ↓Hb (coeliac/CD), U&E (CRF), ESR/CRP (CD), TFTs (hypothyroidism), serum transferrin and pre-albumin concentrations (malnutrition), coeliac screen, IGF1 and IGFBP-3 for GH deficiency.
Stimulation test: glucagon/clonidine to stimulate GH.
Karyotype: genetic conditions.
Sweat test: CF.
X-ray: hand and wrist to assess bone age.
MRI: if neurological symptoms/signs for craniopharyngioma or intracranial tumour.

M: **Referral to paediatric growth specialist:**
Reassurance: for children with familial short stature or constitutional delay.
Treat underlying cause: thyroid hormone in deficient state, optimisation of diet, treatment of underlying chronic disease (coeliac, CF, CD), removal of pituitary tumours.
Growth hormone: licensed indications; GH deficiency, Turner syndrome, renal failure, Prader–Willi syndrome, IUGR (>4 years only). In familial short stature GH treatment does not improve final height (but allows children to reach it sooner), therefore not recommended.
Oxandrolone: low-dose treatment has shown some benefit in improving final height (S/E: high-dose; early fusion of bones so ↓final height)

C: Depends on underlying condition, suggested ↑risk of osteoporosis.

P: **Familial/constitutional short stature:** persists into adulthood; has no effects on life expectancy but may have psychological implications.
GH/thyroid hormone deficiency: can expect to attain height consistent with genetic potential if hormone therapy is started 5 years before puberty.
Chronic disease: final height depends on when treatment of the underlying condition is initiated.

D: Chronic condition with sickling of RBCs caused by production of Hb S instead of Hb A.
Sickle-cell anaemia: homozygous Hb S.
Sickle-cell trait: one copy of Hb S.
Sickle-cell disease: heterozygous Hb S and Hb C, or Hb S and β-thalassaemia.

A: Autosomal recessive inherited point mutation in the β-globin gene, which results in a substitution of valine for glutamic acid on position 6, producing the abnormal protein, Hb S.

A/R: **Precipitating factors:** infection, dehydration, hypoxia, and acidosis.

E: **Sickle-cell anaemia:** 1/1000 live births.
Age of onset: $>$6 months because of continued presence of foetal Hb.
Racial variation: common (5–12%) in African, Caribbean, and Middle-Eastern areas where malaria is prevalent.

H&E: **Thrombotic crisis:**
(1) May mimic acute abdomen.
(2) Acute chest syndrome: SOB, cough, pain, fever.
(3) Severe bony tenderness and swelling especially of the small bones in hands and feet; may cause avascular necrosis which may → infarction and shortened digits.
(4) Persistent erection (priapism); may → impotence.

Aplastic crisis: due to parvovirus that results in temporary cessation of erythropoiesis; characterised by sudden lethargy and pallor.
Sequestration crisis (RBC pooling in spleen/liver): exacerbation of anaemia, hepatomegaly, splenomegaly in early disease with subsequent infarction/autosplenectomy.

P: Hb S polymerises when deoxygenated, resulting in sickling of RBC and ↑fragility and inflexibility. There is ↓RBC survival (~20 days; normal is 120 days) due to sequestration and destruction.

I: **Bloods:** ↓Hb, ↑reticulocytes in haemolytic crisis, ↓reticulocytes in aplastic crisis, U&E, WCC, CRP.
Blood film: sickle cells, anisocytosis, features of hyposplenism (target-cells, Howell–Jolly bodies).
Hb electrophoresis: Hb S, absence of Hb A (in Hb SS), and ↑levels of Hb F.

M: **Acute crisis:** O_2, IV fluids, opiate analgesia, antibiotics.
Infection prophylaxis: penicillin V OD, pneumococcal, meningococcal, Hib vaccination.
Folic acid: for ↑cell turnover.
Hydroxyurea: ↑Hb F levels and ↓frequency and duration of sickle-cell crisis.
RBC transfusion: maintain Hb S level to $<$30%. Iron chelators are required for those who have frequent transfusions.
Exchange transfusion: in sequestration crisis and before surgery.
Advice: nutrition, genetic counselling, antenatal diagnosis.
BMT: in selected patients.
Surgery: joint replacement may be needed for avascular necrosis.

C: ↑Risk of infections with encapsulated organisms, e.g. pneumococcus, *Haemophilus influenzae*, meningococcus, *Salmonella* due to autosplenectomy. Gallstones, renal papillary necrosis, leg ulcers, cardiomyopathy, cerebral infarction.

P: Mortality in children is usually due to infection. With optimal management, patients survive to about 50 years.

D: **Night terrors:** disturbance of the structure of sleep.
Nightmares: repeated episodes of frightening dreams.
Difficulty settling to sleep: child is unable to sleep without parent present.

A: **Night terrors:** fevers, stress, lack of sleep, and medication.
Nightmares: stressful life event, drugs, fever, family history.
Difficulty settling to sleep: separation anxiety.

A/R: **Nightmares:** learning disability, depression, PTSD.

E: **Sleep-related disorders:** one-third of children affected. M = F.
Night terrors: 50% of all infants. Onset usually at ages 4–12 years.
Nightmares: mainly affect ages 3–6 years.
Difficulty settling to sleep: common in toddlers.

H: **Night terrors:**

- Recurrent episodes of intense crying and fear about 1 h 30 min after falling asleep, lasting ~2 min.
- Following night terror, child is difficult to rouse and is disorientated for up to 30 min.
- During night terror child becomes tachypnoeic, tachycardic, and sweats profusely.
- There is no recollection of the episode in the morning.

Nightmares:

- Usually occur in the middle of the night.
- Usually involve a threat to the child, loss of control, or fear of injury.
- The child is highly alert on waking.
- May cause stress and discomfort throughout the day.

E: Usually unremarkable.

P: **Night terrors:** occur during the transition from non-REM sleep to REM sleep with sudden autonomic activation.
Nightmares: occur during REM sleep.

I: None are usually required.
EEG: if associated nocturnal seizures.

M: Parental reassurance. Methods to facilitate better sleeping patterns:
Night terrors:
(1) Ensure the child's sleeping environment is safe.
(2) Regular bedtimes, and remove any possible triggers that could stop the child sleeping.
(3) Keep a record of the times when they occur and wake child shortly before expected night terrors.
Nightmares:
(1) Encourage parents to spend periods of time relaxing with the child.
(2) Psychiatric consultations may be required if there is an underlying stressful event leading to PTSD.
Difficulty settling to sleep:
(1) Routines for sleeping.
(2) In extreme cases sedation for a couple of nights followed by increasing lengths of time between leaving the bedroom and returning, until the child falls asleep in the time that the parent is away.

C: Parental distress and daytime somnolence/anxiety in the child.

P: Night terrors usually occur over a few weeks at a time. Children usually outgrow all sleep disorders.

Slipped upper femoral epiphysis (SUFE)

D: Postero-inferior displacement of femoral head.

A: Unknown. In patients younger than 10 years, a higher association exists for metabolic endocrine disorders:
(1) Hypothyroidism.
(2) Hypogonadism.
(3) Panhypopituitarism.
(4) Renal osteodystrophy.
(5) ↑GH.

A/R: Positive family history (in 5–7% of affected individuals), obesity (places more shear forces around the proximal growth plate in a hip at risk).

E: 1–10/100 000 adolescents.
Peak age: M: 10–16 years, F : 12–14 years.
Sex: M: F = 2.4 : 1.
Adolescents with known unilateral involvement may develop SUFE of the contralateral hip. Left hip > right hip affected.

H: **Acute SUFE:** onset of hip or knee pain, limp, and ↓range of movement within 3 weeks of presentation. Usually occurs after minor injury.
Chronic SUFE: onset of hip or knee pain, limp, and ↓range of movement more than 3 weeks before presentation.

E: **Look:** determine ability to weight bear, and whether there is an antalgic gait. The patient may lie with the foot externally rotated; there may be leg length inequality.
Feel: not so useful in examining the hip (hidden joint).
Move: flexion, abduction, and internal rotation are limited.

P: SUFE results from a Salter–Harris-type growth plate fracture. In adolescents with SUFE, the epiphyseal growth plate is unusually widened. Stress around the hip causes a shear force to be applied to the growth plate, which together with an intrinsic weakness in the cartilage → slipping.

I: **Atypical presentation (age < 10 years):** TFT, LH, FSH, GH, Ca^{2+}, phosphate.
X-ray of pelvis: widening of the growth plate may be seen initially.
AP and lateral X-ray of the hips: radiographic classification is determined by percentage of displacement of the hip in relation to the neck:
Type I (< 33%), Type II (33–50%), and Type III (> 50%).

M: **Paediatric orthopaedic referral:**
Internal fixation: *in situ* central percutaneous pin fixation with one or more cannulated screws. This allows stabilisation of the hip, prevents further slippage, enhances growth plate closure, and alleviates symptoms with minimal morbidity.
Open reduction and internal fixation: chronic slipping may require intracapsular osteotomy for re-alignment once the epiphysis has fused.
Prophylactic treatment of the contralateral hip: may be considered in < 10 years or patients affected by various metabolic endocrine disorders because they have the highest risk of bilateral involvement.

C: Avascular necrosis, chondrolysis (degeneration of articular cartilage), osteoarthritis, leg length inequality.

P: The majority of patients with SUFE do well with *in situ* percutaneous pinning. Patients with a greater degree of slippage (Type III) are at greater risk of developing complications.

Sticky eyes in the neonate

D: **Sticky eyes in the newborn:** may have non-infectious cause (blocked tear duct) or infectious cause (see **A**) which may or may not be associated with a purulent discharge.

A: (1) *Staphylococcus aureus, Streptococcus pneumoniae, Strep. viridans,* and *Staph. epidermidis.*

(2) *Chlamydia trachomatis* is the most common; its reservoir is the maternal cervix or urethra.

(3) *Neisseria gonorrhoea* is a gram-negative diplococcus, which is potentially the most dangerous and virulent infectious cause.

A/R: Maternal genital chlamydia or gonococcal infection.

E: 1% live births.

H&E: **Staphylococcal/Streptococcal organisms:** mild presentation; may present with lid oedema, conjunctival injection, chemosis (swelling/oedema of the conjunctiva), and/or discharge.

Gonococcal: usually presents on day 1.

Classical presentation: bilateral purulent conjunctivitis, associated with marked lid oedema and chemosis. The cornea may become ulcerated and can → perforation.

Extraocular involvement: rhinitis, stomatitis, arthritis, and meningitis may also be present.

Chlamydial: the incubation period is 5–14 days. Presentation ranges from mild hyperaemia with scant mucoid discharge to lid swelling chemosis and pseudomembrane formation. Rarely, blindness can be caused by eyelid scarring and pannus (infiltration of the cornea with blood vessels).

Extraocular involvement: pneumonitis, otitis, pharyngeal and rectal colonisation.

Other microbial agents: usually milder presentation; may present with lid oedema, conjunctival injection, chemosis, and/or discharge.

P: The conjunctiva is a mucous membrane that forms the outermost layer of the eye. Any type of irritation to the eye causes vasodilation of the conjunctival blood vessels, giving the typical red appearance as well as chemosis and excessive secretions. The reaction is more severe in the neonate because of lack of immunity, absence of lymphoid tissue, and absence of tears at birth.

I: **Microsopy, culture and sensitivity:** bacterial swab of any discharge.

Chlamydial culture: if treatment is contemplated prior to results, a chlamydia swab should also be taken and sent in virus transport medium.

M: **Preliminary empirical treatment:** neomycin or tetracycline eye drops or ointment.

(1) Staphylococcal/Streptococcal organisms: chloramphenicol eye drops.

(2) *N. gonorrhoea*: third-generation cephalosporin IV.

(3) Chlamydial infection: tetracycline eye drops and oral erythromycin to protect against pneumonia.

Prevention: antenatal treatment of maternal and paternal STDs.

Notification: chlamydia and gonorrhoea are notifiable diseases (CCDC).

C: Iritis, corneal scarring +/− perforation, blindness, extraocular manifestations of chlamydial and gonococcal infection.

P: Infants who develop conjunctivitis are generally detected very early and treated promptly; therefore there is an excellent prognosis.

D: The sudden death of an infant under 1 year of age that remains unexplained after a thorough case investigation, including performance of a complete post-mortem, examination of the death scene, and a review of the clinical history (National Institute of Child Health and Development).

A: There are multiple factors that have been implicated in SIDS; however, none have been proven:

Prolonged QT interval: is a marker of reduced cardiac electrical stability and is strongly associated with SIDS. 30–35% of infants who die of SIDS are estimated to have prolonged QT interval in the 1st week of life. An ↑ in sympathetic activity in these infants may be sufficient to cause fatal arrhythmias such as torsades de points.

Upper airways obstruction:
(1) Developing infants have sites of anatomical and physiological vulnerability such as a shallow hypopharynx and position of the tongue and epiglottis.
(2) Infants are obligate nasal breathers for the first few months of life and so prone positioning may compress their only airway.

Central apnoea: infants can have reflex-like apnoeic responses to a number of conditions such as hypoxia, hypoglycaemia, infection and stimulation of the upper larynx (e.g. GOR). Such apnoeic responses are probably due to incomplete development of the CNS, ↑vagal tone, and ↓respiratory muscle reserve.

Thermoregulatory dysfunction: minor changes in temperature (hot or cold) can induce autonomic dysfunction in infants.

Brainstem dysfunction: cardiorespiratory function, autonomic mechanisms, chemoreceptor sensitivity, and thermoregulation are all controlled by the medullary and related structures of the brain. Autopsy examinations of the brainstems of infants with a diagnosis of SIDS have demonstrated hypoplasia or ↓neurotransmitter binding of the arcuate nucleus.

A/R: **Acute life-threatening events:** characterised by some combination of apnoea (central, occasionally obstructive), colour change (usually cyanotic or pallid), hypotonia, choking, or gagging. Survivors of an acute life-threatening event share many risk factors for SIDS and are at a significantly ↑risk.

Risk factors: preterm infants, sleeping prone, overheating, maternal drug abuse/smoking during pregnancy, low socio-economic status, family members who smoke, bottlefed rather than breastfed infants, young maternal age (< 20 years).

E: SIDS is the most common cause of death in infants aged 1 month to 1 year.

Peak incidence: 1–4 months.

Incidence: 1.7 cases/1000 live births. Occurs during hours of extended sleep (10 PM to 10 AM).

Seasonal variation: more common during winter.

Sex: M > F.

H&E: SIDS is a diagnosis of exclusion; therefore a thorough history describing the details surrounding the event and examination is required to look for possible medical conditions leading to demise.

Classical presentation:
(1) Child is found dead usually in the position the child was put to bed.
(2) Checks whilst the child was asleep usually revealed no problems.
(3) Parent may report that the child 'was not himself or herself' before going to sleep.
(4) May report GI or respiratory infection in the weeks preceding death.

Alerts for child abuse: unclear, inconsistent history, unwanted child, poor antenatal/postnatal care, previous SIDS infant under same carer, age > 6 months. See Child abuse for examination.

P: See **A**.

I: Post-mortem examination.

M: Provide support and a calm environment for the family.
Allow both parents to spend time with the child, allow photographs if desired.
Avoid mention of risk factors which attribute blame.
SIDS support groups.
Prevention:
(1) Avoid smoking during pregnancy and by family members following birth.
(2) Avoid overheating the baby, e.g. with duvets, use thin flat sheets that are firmly fastened and will not cover the baby's head.
(3) Place the baby in the supine position; 'back to sleep' campaign reduced incidence of SIDS significantly in the UK.
(4) Use of firm flat bedding; infants are more likely to sleep face down with soft bedding.

C: Psychological distress in family members.

P: N/A.

D: Arrhythmia of the heart's rhythm and rate characterised by tachycardia.

A: SVTs involve components of the conduction system within or above the bundle of His.

3 major categories:

- Re-entrant tachycardia using an accessory pathway such as WPW syndrome.
- Re-entrant tachycardia without an accessory pathway such as AV node re-entry tachycardia or atrial flutter.
- Ectopic atrial tachycardia or ↑automaticity.

A/R: Electrolyte and acid–base disturbances.

E: 2.25/1000 children.

H&E: **General:** characterised by sudden onset and resolution. May be precipitated by an acute infection and usually occurs when the patient is at rest.

Children: HR ranges from 180 to 300 bpm. Palpitations may be the only complaint. Many children tolerate these attacks very well; only exceptionally rapid rates or prolonged attacks progress to heart failure.

Young infants: more obscure diagnosis as HR is normally rapid and communication of symptoms is difficult. HR ranges from 200 to 300 bpm. Usual presentation is with heart failure.

The infant may become acutely ill in attacks lasting >6 h with ashen complexion and irritability.

Neonates: differentiation from sinus tachycardia is difficult, but if the HR is invariable, abnormal P-wave axis is present and HR >230 bpm, SVT should be suspected.

P: **Re-entrant tachycardia using an accessory pathway:**

- Initiated by a premature atrial beat that is most often conducted to the ventricle through the normal AV nodal pathway.
- The ventricular response finds the AV nodal pathway refractory, but the bypass tract readily conducts in a retrograde fashion, hence it returns to the atrium as an echo beat.
- This echo beat is then transmitted to the ventricle and the cycle repeats itself.

I: **ECG:** narrow complex tachycardia. With severe heart failure there may be myocardial ischaemic changes (T-wave inversion in the lateral precordial leads).

WPW syndrome: characteristic features are usually seen when the patient is not experiencing tachycardia; short PR interval and slow upstroke of the QRS (δ wave).

M: **Medical conversion to sinus rhythm:**

(1) Vagotonic manoeuvres: Valsalva manoeuvre, submersion of the face in iced saline, breath-holding or carotid sinus massage.

(2) IV adenosine is the treatment of choice in the acute situation and induces AV block, hence terminating the re-entry circuit.

(3) Synchronised DC cardioversion may be used if treatment with adenosine fails or if the child is compromised.

Recurrent SVTs: accessory pathways are usually identified and ablated.

C: Hydrops foetalis, severe heart failure.

P: Patients with symptomatic WPW syndrome have a small risk of sudden death. Otherwise, patients with SVT in the setting of a structurally normal heart have an excellent prognosis.

Testicular torsion

D: The testicle twists on the spermatic cord, occluding its blood supply from the testicular artery.

A: **Intravaginal torsion:** the typical testicle is covered by the tunica vaginalis, which attaches to the posterolateral surface of the testicle and allows for little mobility. Torsion may be idiopathic or due to the congenital bell clapper deformity (12% of cases). In this condition patients have an inappropriately high attachment of the tunica vaginalis, so the testis can rotate freely on the spermatic cord within the tunica vaginalis.
Extravaginal torsion (5%): develops antenatally in the spermatic cord, proximal to the attachments of the tunica vaginalis.

A/R: **DD:**
Torsion of testicular appendage (hydatid of Morgagni):
(1) Occurs a little earlier (7–12 years).
(2) Causes less pain (patient can walk without pain).
Epididymitis, orchitis, epididymo-orchitis:
(1) Occurs in older patients and onset of pain is gradual and usually associated with dysuria.
(2) Commonly 2° to reflux from UTI or STD *(gonococcus, chlamydia).*
(3) May be 2° to an underlying congenital, acquired, structural, or urologic abnormality.
Hydrocele: painless swelling that transilluminates.
Testicular tumour: insidious onset of scrotal enlargement, usually painless.
Idiopathic scrotal oedema: scrotal skin is thickened, oedematous, and often inflamed. The testis is not tender and is of normal size and position.
Acute appendicitis: torsion may mimic an acute abdomen.

E: 1/4000 boys. L > R. Bilateral in 2%.
Peak age intravaginal torsion: 14 years (range 11–30 years).

H&E: **Extravaginal torsion:** manifests as a firm, hard, scrotal mass. The scrotal skin characteristically fixes to the necrotic testis.
Intravaginal torsion:
(1) Sudden onset of severe unilateral scrotal pain followed by scrotal swelling and erythema.
(2) Hard and tender testicle tends to lie high and horizontally in comparison to the other testis.
(3) May have a history of prior episodes of intermittent testicular pain that has resolved spontaneously (intermittent torsion and detorsion).
(4) May be associated with nausea and vomiting, abdominal pain, fever, urinary frequency.

P: Twisting of the testicle on the spermatic cord → venous occlusion and engorgement, with subsequent arterial ischaemia causing infarction of the testicle.

I: **Diagnosis is clinical.**
Doppler USS: may demonstrate reduced/absent blood flow and differentiate from epididymitis but must not delay surgery.

M: **Surgical emergency:** torsion must be relieved in <6 h for the testis to remain viable.
Orchidopexy: if the testis is viable, it is untwisted and fixed to the scrotum. The contralateral testis should be fixed at the same time.
Orchidectomy: if the testis is not viable. Testicular prostheses are available.

C: Delayed diagnosis or treatment may result in a non-viable testis.

P: Good if emergency surgery is performed without delay.

D: Cyanotic CHD, which consists of 4 structural defects to the heart:
(1) Large VSD.
(2) Infundibular and valvular pulmonary stenosis.
(3) RVH.
(4) Overriding of the aorta with respect to the ventricular septum (aorta sits on top of VSD).

A: Complex anatomical abnormalities arising from the abnormal development of the right ventricular infundibulum.

A/R: Foetal hydantoin, foetal carbamazepine, FAS, Down syndrome.

E: 5/10 000 live births.

H&E: **Neonatal:** if there is pulmonary atresia, child becomes cyanosed when the ductus arteriosus closes.
Infants:
- Hypoxic 'spells' give rise to pallor or cyanosis with respiratory distress.
- Harsh ejection systolic murmur at left sternal edge/pulmonary area, which radiates to the back.
- Loud single 2nd heart sound due to loss of the pulmonary valve.
- Parasternal thrust in RVH.

Older children:
- Often adopt a squatting position with 'spells'.

This improves symptoms by two means:
(1) Squatting ↑ systemic vascular resistance and thereby decreases the right → left shunt through the large VSD.
(2) Squatting ↑ systemic venous return which improves blood flow to the pulmonary system and ↑ blood oxygenation.
- May exhibit signs of CHF.

P: **Severity of disease is determined by degree of pulmonary outflow tract obstruction.** This results in:
(1) Reduced blood flow into lungs.
(2) Elevation of right ventricular pressure → RVH.
(3) Resistance to ejection into the pulmonary circulation produces right → left shunting through the large VSD and deoxygenated blood going back into the systemic circulation.

Hypoxic spells: due to ↑right → left shunting, which results in a reduction in pulmonary flow. It is thought to be due to infundibular spasm.

I: **CXR:** normal/small-shaped heart with uptilted apex 2° to RVH and concave pulmonary segment, which in severe cases appears 'boot-shaped'. Dark lungs due to reduced lung vascularity reflects ↓pulmonary flow.
ECG: right axis deviation and evidence of RVH.
Bloods: ↑Hb (polycythaemia 2° to hypoxia).
Echo: confirms diagnosis.

M: **Treatment of cyanotic spells:** soothe the distressed infant to try and induce sleep. If prolonged (> 15 min), they require treatment with pain relief, sedation (e.g. morphine) and IV propanolol.
Corrective surgical intervention: carried out in early infancy to widen the pulmonary valve and close the VSD.

C: (1) Hypoxic attacks can result in myocardial infarction, cerebrovascular accidents, and death.
(2) 2° polycythaemia may → cerebral thromboembolic events.
(3) Infective endocarditis.
(4) Cerebral abscess.
(5) Delayed growth and development.

P: Pre-surgery 30% mortality in the 1st year of life and 75% by 10 years. With surgery now 90% survive to adult life and 90% of these have a normal lifestyle.

Thalassaemia

D: Heterogeneous group of autosomal recessive defects of globin synthesis.

A: **β-thalassaemia major:** homozygous point mutations/deletions in the β-globin genes on chromosome 11 $\rightarrow \beta^0$ (no β-chains)/β^+ (small amounts).
β-thalassaemia trait: asymptomatic heterozygous carriers, mild microcytic hypochromic anaemia; may be confused with iron deficiency anaemia.
β-thalassaemia intermedia: several different gene defects cause mild β-globin synthesis abnormalities with variable clinical features, symptomatic anaemia, hepatosplenomegaly, and extramedullary haemopoiesis.
α-thalassaemia: $\downarrow\alpha$-globin chain synthesis. There are 4 α-globin genes on chromosome 16. Severity of disease depends on number of genes deleted.

A/R: Due to geographical distribution individuals affected may also inherit sickle cell gene.

E: Common in Mediterranean, Middle-Eastern, and SE Asian populations. There has been a marked reduction due to antenatal diagnosis and termination of pregnancy.

H: Anaemia and jaundice at 3–6 months (when γ-chain synthesis switches to β-chain synthesis), failure to thrive, recurrent infections.

E: Pallor, jaundice, frontal bossing, and maxillary overgrowth due to marrow hyperplasia and hepatosplenomegaly due to haemolysis, extramedullary haemopoiesis and iron overload.

P: Reduced synthesis of β-globin chain $\rightarrow$ excess of other chains $\rightarrow$ precipitation of erythroblasts and erythrocytes in the bone marrow $\rightarrow$ ineffective erythropoiesis, haemolysis, anaemia, and extramedullary haemopoiesis.

I: **Bloods:** $\downarrow$Hb, $\downarrow$MCV, $\downarrow$MCH. **Film:** target cells, nucleated RBCs, $\uparrow$reticulocytes.
Skull X-ray: hair-on-end appearance due to expansion of bone marrow into the cortex.
Hb electrophoresis: absent/$\downarrow$HbA and $\uparrow$HbF($\alpha_2\gamma_2$), $\uparrow$HbA$_2$($\alpha_2\delta_2$) as γ and δ chain production continues.
Bone marrow: hypercellular with erythroid hyperplasia.
DNA analysis: for specific mutations (antenatal and postnatal CVS)

M: **Medical:** blood transfusions (maintain Hb > 10 g/dl), iron chelation with desferrioxamine, vitamin C ($\uparrow$iron excretion), hepatitis B immunisation.
Surgical: splenectomy after 6 years to $\downarrow$blood requirements:

- Before splenectomy: pneumococcus/meningococcus/*Haemophilus influenzae* vaccinations.
- After splenectomy: daily penicillin, low-dose aspirin for post-splenectomy thrombocytosis to $\downarrow$risk of thromboembolism.

BMT: from HLA-matching sibling, 90% success rate.

C: **Iron overload:** 'slate-grey' skin pigmentation ($\uparrow$melanin and haemosiderin), cirrhosis, hepatoma, short stature, delayed puberty, DM, hypothyroidism, hypoparathyroidism, cardiomyopathy.
Antibody formation: RBC antibodies, HLA antibodies.
Infections: meningococcal and pneumococcal after splenectomy, *Yersinia enterocolitica* in those taking desferrioxamine.
Osteoporosis: 2° to marrow expansion and endocrinological complications.
Hypersplenism: leads to $\downarrow$Hb, $\downarrow$Plt, $\downarrow$neutrophils.

P: Good with regular transfusion and iron chelation. Mortality is mainly due to infections and heart failure in untreated iron overload. Without transfusions β-thalassaemia major is fatal.

Tics

D: **Tics:** stereotyped movements of muscle groups that have no useful function.
Tourette syndrome: chronic idiopathic syndrome with both motor and vocal tics beginning before adulthood.

A: **Genetic:** suggested by significantly higher concordance in monozygotic twins compared to dizygotic twins, and significantly higher incidence in 1st degree relatives of sufferers.
Acquired: there is a possible subgroup who have antibodies to β-haemolytic streptococci that crossreact with neurons.

A/R: ADHD in > 30%, OCD in > 20%.

E: **Tic disorders:** 3–15% of children according to different studies, declining to 2–3% by adolescence.
Tourette syndrome: 0.5–1%. M : F = 2 : 1.

H&E: **Simple tics:** brief movements involving few muscle groups, e.g. eye blinking, shoulder shrugging, clearing the throat, and humming.
Complex tics: coordinated patterns of successive movements involving several muscle groups, e.g. jumping, touching the nose, echolalia (repeating another's speech), and coprolalia (outbursts of obscenities).
Tics are worsened by stress and reduced by absorbing activities, markedly reduced during sleep and suppressible for brief periods of time.
Tourette syndrome: multiple motor and vocal tics occur (not necessarily concurrently). Tics occur many times a day, nearly every day for more than 1 year and frequently vary in nature, severity, and location. *Rage attacks* consist of explosive, unpredictable outbursts out of proportion to stimuli threatening destruction and self-injury, followed by immediate remorse.

P: Unknown. Theories include a reduction in the basal ganglia's inhibition of undesired motor programmes.

I: **Usually none required.**
In specific cases investigations may be appropriate to exclude organic cause:
(1) Anti-streptolysin titre, especially if there was sudden onset of tics post impetigo, pharyngitis, or otitis media.
(2) TFTs to exclude hyperthyroidism.
(3) Serum caeruloplasmin to exclude Wilson disease.
(4) EEG to assess for absence seizures.
To assess for comorbid psychiatric disease: psychometric testing and MSE for ADHD and OCD.

M: **Multidisciplinary team approach:**
Supportive: parental education and notify school of diagnosis.
Behavioural therapy: habit reversal.
Medical treatment: neuroleptic drugs (lower dose than for psychosis), dopamine agonists.
Treatment of comorbid psychiatric disease:
(1) OCD: SSRIs.
(2) ADHD: tricyclic antidepressants (psychostimulants such as methylphenidate used in treating ADHD can cause tics).

C: Stigma associated with outbursts may → social withdrawal. Interruption in thought and conversation affects education. Self-injurious behaviour may arise from depression.

P: Tics can progressively worsen in childhood but abate or diminish markedly by the age of 18 in 90% of cases. There is significant morbidity associated with comorbid psychiatric disease.

D: Symptomatic congenital infection with *Toxoplasma gondii.*

A: **Transplacental transmission:**

- Occurs in 40% of mothers who have active 1° infection. They may contract this from eating undercooked poultry, handling cat litter, or from blood transfusions.
- Latent toxoplasmosis may reactivate in women with HIV and result in congenital transmission.
- Risk of transmission is greatest in the 3rd trimester.
- The severity of infection in the foetus depends on the gestational age at the time of transmission.

Postnatal transmission: infants usually contract a much milder form of the disease.

A/R: Undercooked meat, handling cat litter, immunocompromise.

E: 1/10 000 live births.

H&E: **Mother:** 1° infection in an otherwise healthy mother can be asymptomatic or mild; with malaise, painless lymphadenopathy (usually cervical), myalgia, and a low-grade fever.

1st trimester infections: may result in foetal death *in utero* or in the neonate with severe CNS involvement, such as cerebral calcifications and hydrocephalus.

2nd–3rd trimester infections: infants are usually asymptomatic at birth and subsequently may develop the following sequelae:

- **Eyes:** chorioretinitis with diplopia, scotoma, and/or photophobia.
- **Neurological:** nystagmus, hypertonicity, and/or seizures.
- **Others:** jaundice, hepatomegaly, splenomegaly, rash, lymphadenopathy, bulging fontanelle, micro/macrocephaly.

P: *T. gondii* is an intracellular protozoan. Lymph nodes typically show reactive follicular hyperplasia as well as irregular groups of histiocytes around the edges of the germinal centres.

I: **Antenatal diagnosis:**

20–24 week USS: in severe infection the foetus may exhibit hydrocephalus.

Cordocentisis: to confirm foetal infection during early pregnancy.

Neonatal diagnosis:

Serology: persistent or rising IgG titres indicate active infection rather than maternal antibodies.

Sabin–Feldman dye test: measures IgG antibodies.

CT/MRI brain: in cerebral toxoplasmosis there are multiple ring-enhancing lesions.

M: **Detection during pregnancy:** counselling, consider termination of pregnancy or introduction of spiramycin.

Prevention: avoid eating undercooked poultry, unpasteurised milk, and uncooked eggs, wear gloves when handling cat litter during pregnancy.

Infant: 1-year course of pyrimethamine with folic acid supplements, clindamycin.

C: **Ophthalmic:** the asymptomatic infant is at risk of chorioretinitis during adulthood, and subsequent blindness.

Neurological: hydrocephalus, cerebral calcifications, seizures.

P: Neonates who are symptomatic at birth often die in the 1st month of life. Infants with severe infection may have persistent hearing and visual impairment and learning disability. Immunocompromised children have a higher morbidity and mortality.

Transient synovitis (TS)/Irritable hip

D: Arthralgia and arthritis 2° to a transient inflammation of the synovium of the hip.

A: Ligamentous or minor capsular injury.

A/R: **Associated:** recent URTI (in 50% of children with TS).
Related: juvenile arthritis, arthritis associated with inflammatory bowel disease, psoriasis and ankylosing spondylitis, reactive arthritis from *Campylobacter*, *Salmonella*, and *Shigella*.

E: Commonest cause of acute hip pain in children aged 2–12 years.
Sex: M : F = 2 : 1.

H: Elicit history of trauma, previous URTI, previous episodes of TS.

General: well-looking child; toxic-looking child is more likely to have septic arthritis.
Pain: onset over hours to days. Unilateral hip or groin pain is common, may have radiation to the knee or medial thigh on movement. Usually no pain at rest.
Limp: child may present with a painless limp or antalgic gait and complain of pain while walking.
Fever: unusual; may have mild fever ($< 38°C$), if any higher, then septic arthritis must be considered.

E: **Look:** leg may be held in flexion and internal rotation, no leg length inequality (differentiate from other causes of a limping child).
Feel: hip may be tender to palpation.
Move: mild restriction in range of movement, particularly internal rotation and abduction.
Leg roll: patient is supine whilst involved leg is rolled from side to side – involuntary muscle guarding occurs on one side when compared to the other.

P: Non-specific inflammation, hypertrophy of synovial membrane, ↑proteoglycans in the synovial fluid.

I: **Bloods:** CRP/ESR normal or slightly ↑, WCC normal or slightly ↑.
Blood culture: negative. **Urine culture:** negative.
AP and lateral X-ray of the pelvis: medial joint space may be slightly wider in the affected hip. Half to two-thirds of patients with TS may have an accentuated pericapsular shadow. Look for signs of SUFE or LCPD (see chapters).
USS: small joint effusion with bulging of anterior joint capsule.
Joint aspiration: under USS guidance only if septic arthritis is suspected.

M: Once septic arthritis is excluded, management is supportive; avoid weight bearing on the affected limb, analgesia with NSAIDs.

In severe cases refer to paediatric orthopaedic surgeon for skin traction with the hip in 45° flexion.

C: May be the initial presentation of LCPD (develops in 1.5% of children with TS) or SUFE.

P: Improves within days. Most have complete resolution in 2 weeks.

Recurs in up to 15%, mostly within 6 months.

D: Acute, self-limiting tachypnoea in the absence of other cause such as metabolic acidosis, RDS, or infection.

A: Infants almost invariably recover fully; therefore it is difficult to define TTN pathologically.
Hypothesis: thought to be due to delayed resorption of foetal lung fluid. The delayed resorption causes ↓pulmonary compliance and ↓tidal volume with ↑dead space.

A/R: TTN is more common after elective Caesarean section and precipitous deliveries. This is thought to be due to ↓time in labour. Lung liquid is predominately reabsorbed actively by pneumocytes (type I) as a result of the changes in hormones, and prostaglandins during labour. If there is no time for this to occur, the fluid is not reabsorbed.

E: Commonest cause of respiratory distress in full-term infants.
1–2% of newborn infants have respiratory distress; of these 33–50% have TTN. Other causes: RDS, metabolic acidosis, congenital cardiac disorders.

H: **Onset:** usually occurs in the first 1–3 h following an uneventful normal preterm, term vaginal, or elective Caesarean section delivery.
Duration: most cases resolve within 24–36 h.

E: Early onset of tachypnoea in the neonate; may also display signs of respiratory distress such as recession; intercostal/subcostal/sternal expiratory grunting, nasal flaring and in severe cases cyanosis.

P: Prominent perihilar streaking seen on CXR is usually the result of engorgement of the periarterial lymphatics that participate in the clearance of the alveolar fluid.

I: **CXR:** prominent perihilar streaking, patchy infiltrates, fluid in the horizontal fissure, flat diaphragms, and occasional pleural fluid.
ABG: degree of ↓pO_2 depends on the amount of fluid on the lungs.
Blood culture: to exclude infectious cause of respiratory distress.

M: It is important to exclude other causes of neonatal respiratory distress such as pneumonia (e.g. group B haemolytic streptococcus), meconium aspiration, pulmonary haemorrhage, or cerebral hyperventilation that follows birth asphyxia.
Management: continual monitoring and supportive care.
(1) Ventilatory support as required including supplemental oxygen and occasionally CPAP.
(2) Maintenance hydration and dextrose IV.
(3) Feeds should be withheld until respiratory rate < 60/min to reduce likelihood of aspiration.
(4) Empirical antibiotics. Discontinue once infectious cause of RDS has been excluded (negative cultures).

C: Usually no complications if managed with good supportive measures.

P: Excellent.

Transposition of the great arteries (TGA)

D: Cyanotic CHD with transposition of the aorta and the PA.

A: Embryology likely to involve abnormal persistence of the subaortic conus with resorption or underdevelopment of the subpulmonary conus (infundibulum). This abnormality aligns the aorta anterior and superior to the right ventricle during development.

A/R: Maternal rubella, poor antenatal nutrition, FAS, maternal age >40 years and maternal DM.

E: 2/10 000 live births. M : F = 3 : 2.

H&E: Depends on the extent of intercirculatory mixing and the presence of associated anatomic lesions.

(1) **TGA with intact ventricular septum:** prominent and progressive cyanosis within <24 h.
(2) **TGA with large VSD:** infants may be asymptomatic initially or may exhibit mild cyanosis when crying. Parasternal heave 2° to RVH. In the first 3–6 weeks infant may exhibit signs of CHF as pulmonary blood flow increases.
(3) **TGA with VSD and left ventricular (pulmonary) outflow tract obstruction:** patients present in a similar fashion to tetralogy of Fallot.
(4) **TGA with VSD and pulmonary vascular obstructive disease:** patients present with progressive cyanosis, despite early balloon atrial septostomy.

P: Circulations are in parallel instead of in series. Results in systemic (deoxygenated) blood recirculating through the body, and pulmonary (oxygenated) blood recirculating through the lungs. Survival is reliant on transfer of blood from each circuit into the other via a patent foramen ovale, PDA, or ASD/VSD.

I: **CXR:** narrow mediastinum due to AP relationship of the great vessels, ↑pulmonary vascular markings due to ↑pulmonary flow. In severe cases 'egg-shaped' heart due to the hypertrophied right ventricle.
Echo: diagnostic.

M: **Medical:** pre-op correction of electrolyte abnormalities and a prostaglandin infusion to maintain patency of the ductus arteriosus.
Radiological intervention: balloon atrial septostomy is performed by passing a catheter with an expandable balloon at its tip into the left atrium via the right atrium and foramen ovale. The balloon is inflated within the left atrium and then pulled through the atrial septum. This tears the atrial septum, so allowing mixing of the systemic and pulmonary venous blood within the atrium.
Surgical: subsequent 'arterial switch procedure' is performed in the first few weeks of life. The PA and aorta are transected above the arterial valves and switched over. The coronary arteries are also transferred across to the new aorta.

C: CHF, cardiac arrhythmias, progressive pulmonary hypertension, polycythaemia 2° to prolonged hypoxia.

P: The mortality rate in untreated patients is ~30% in the 1st week, 50% in the 1st month, and 90% by the end of the 1st year. The overall survival rate following arterial switch operation is 90%.

D: Genetic defect of the sex chromosomes in females resulting in the majority of individuals having the karyotype 45XO.

A: 50% of affected individuals have only one X chromosome (45XO). Other defects include a deletion of the short arm of one X chromosome resulting in an isochromosome with 2 long arms and no short arms. Others include the mosaic 45X/46XX and rarely 45X/46XY. Inheritance is sporadic.

A/R: Not associated with ↑maternal age.

E: 1/2500 live births.

H: **Antenatal:** >95%, which results in early miscarriage.
Childhood: secretory otitis media in 50%, which results in conductive hearing loss.
Adolescence: ovarian dysgenesis, which results in infertility in later life.

E: **Congenital malformations:** congenital heart defects (20%), especially COA, horseshoe kidney (40%), and ovarian dysgenesis (95%).

Physical signs: neonatal lymphoedema of the hand and feet, neck webbing, wide carrying angle (cubitus valgus), widely spaced nipples, pigmented naevi, and short 4th metacarpal.

Growth and development:

(1) Normal intellectual development (low average).
(2) Short stature (however, growth is normal for 4 years until the ovaries involute), Turner growth charts are available.

P: Webbed neck is caused by the cystic hygroma of the neck in early foetal life.

I: **Antenatal:** is occasionally detected with antenatal ultrasound investigation due to presence of a cystic hygroma or foetal oedema of the neck.
Amniocentesis and chromosomal analysis can be performed to confirm/exclude diagnosis.
Chromosomal studies: patients have a characteristic appearance, but diagnosis is from karyotype analysis as patients with Noonan syndrome are phenotypically very similar to patients with Turner syndrome.

M: **Management is of the individual symptoms:**
Surgical treatment:

(1) Congenital heart defects.
(2) Grommets may be inserted if secretory otitis media causes significant hearing loss.
(3) Plastic surgery for the neck webbing.
(4) Removal of gonads if present as 50% become neoplastic.

Hormonal treatment:

(1) Treatment with GH from mid-childhood to ↑ final height.
(2) The gradual introduction of oestrogen replacement in early adolescence promotes the development of 2° sexual characteristics.

C: Most patients with Turner syndrome remain infertile despite oestrogen replacement therapy. Gonads may be present if there is a Y chromosome present (mosaic).

P: Good with treatment options available; patients can expect to have a normal lifespan.

Upper respiratory tract infection (URTI)

D: A number of different conditions such as the common cold (coryza), sore throat (pharyngitis and tonsillitis), and middle ear infection (otitis media).

A: Viruses cause $>$90% of URTIs.
Coryza: rhinovirus, coronavirus, RSV.
Pharyngitis: adenovirus, enterovirus, rhinovirus, group A β-haemolytic streptococcus in older children.
Tonsillitis: EBV causing infectious mononucleosis, group A β-haemolytic streptococcus.
Otitis media: influenza, parainfluenza, enteroviruses and adenovirus, streptococcus pneumoniae, non-typeable *Haemophilus influenzae* (i.e. not Hib), *Moraxella catarrhalis*.
Underimmunised child: *Corynebacterium diphtheriae* is a severe, life-threatening cause of pharyngitis and tonsillitis.

A/R: M $>$ F, URTIs are universally prevalent and are not associated with factors associated with low socio-economic class (e.g. household smoking) as are LRTIs.

E: Very common. 2 peaks: starting nursery (2–3 years) and starting primary school (4–5 years).

H: **General:** lethargy, poor feeding.
Coryza: sneezing, sore throat, fever is variable.
Pharyngitis/tonsillitis: fever, sore throat, cough, abdominal pain; mesenteric adenitis is often preceded by a URTI with subsequent enlargement of the mesenteric lymph nodes.
Infectious mononucleosis: prolonged lethargy, malaise, sore throat.
Otitis media: ear pain; infant may scream and pull at ear, conductive hearing loss in chronic secretory otitis media.

E: **General:** toxicity, pyrexia, tachycardia, cervical lymphadenopathy.
Coryza: nasal discharge (rhinitis).
Pharyngitis: the pharynx, soft palate, and tonsillar fauces are inflamed and swollen.
Tonsillitis: red, swollen tonsils with or without white exudates. Follicular tonsillitis with white exudates may be due to adenovirus, EBV, or group A β-haemolytic streptococcus.
Otitis media: tympanic membranes bright red and bulging on otoscopy with loss of normal light reflex.

P: **Macro:** reactive inflammation of the URT to infectious agent with production of serous fluid (rhinitis) and swelling of mucosal lining.

I: **Throat swab:** may grow Group A β-haemolytic streptococcus. Used in complicated tonsillitis/pharyngitis to rule out diphtheria.
Bloods: ASOT, monospot test (EBV).

M: **Treat pyrexia:** regular paracetamol +/− ibuprofen may be required to bring down temperature. Especially important if the child is prone to febrile convulsions. Do not use aspirin as may precipitate Reye's syndrome (severe liver disease).
Active treatment: oral antibiotics such as penicillin or erythromycin (if penicillin-allergic) for 10 days to prevent rheumatic fever are indicated if group A β-haemolytic streptococcus grows on throat swab.
Surgical intervention: tonsillectomy is rarely indicated, only when recurrent tonsillitis is causing significant loss of schooling or upper airways obstruction and sleep apnoea.

C: (1) Recurrent acute tonsillitis/tonsillar hypertrophy.
(2) Peritonsillar abscess: *Quinsy*.
(3) Post-streptococcal immunological response, e.g. acute GN.

P: **Excellent; duration of illness 1–2 weeks.**
'Treat a cold it lasts a week, don't treat and it lasts 7 days.'

D: Congenital structural abnormalities of the kidneys.

A: Majority are congenital or inherited defects:

(1) **Infantile polycystic kidney disease:** autosomal recessive disorder, which causes multiple cysts in the renal cortex and medulla. The majority also have liver cysts.
(2) **Medullary sponge kidney:** inherited condition causing cystic dilation of the collecting ducts, which allows formation of calculi in these ducts.
(3) **Nephronophthisis:** autosomal dominant or recessive defect causing multiple cyst formation at the corticomedullary junction with progressive glomerular sclerosis.
(4) **Unilateral renal agenesis:** congenital.
(5) **Ectopic/horseshoe kidney:** congenital.

A/R: Associated with other congenital malformations (cardiac, pulmonary, cleft palate, CNS).

E: **Infantile polycystic kidney disease:** 1–4/10 000 live births. M = F.
Medullary sponge kidney: 1–4/20 000 live births. The rest are very rare.

H&E: **Antenatal presentation:** renal agenesis, horseshoe kidney, and infantile polycystic disease can present antenatally with oligohydramnios due to ↓foetal urine output. In severe cases this results in pulmonary hypoplasia and most of these infants die from pulmonary complications shortly after birth.
Infantile polycystic kidney disease: bilateral flank masses are usually detected at birth. If the diagnosis is missed in the neonatal period, children may present with haematuria, hypertension, hepatosplenomegaly, and failure to thrive. Older children and adolescents may present with complications from liver fibrosis such as a GI bleed from oesophageal varices.
Medullary sponge kidney: predisposed to UTIs and renal calculi.
Nephronophthisis: usually presents at age 4–6 with polyuria, 2° enuresis and polydipsia.
Ectopic renal masses: may be palpable in the pelvis.
Horseshoe kidney: may be palpable as a midline mass with transmitted aortic pulsation.

P: Abnormal renal position and tissue are usually visually apparent. Kidney(s) may be enlarged, shrunken, absent, or displaced. Presence of cysts may be visible through the renal capsule. Intrarenal calculi are common in medullary sponge kidney.

I: **USS:** effective and non-invasive.
IVU: allows visualisation of ectopic kidneys and medullary 'blush' in sponge kidneys.
Nuclear renal imaging: DTPA, DMSA, and MAG3 are common radio-labelled agents used for assessment of kidney function and perfusion.

M: **Advice:** patient education and genetic counselling.
Of hypertension: ACE inhibitors, Ca^{2+} channel blockers, β-blockers, and diuretics.
Of renal osteodystrophy: calcium supplements, phosphate binders, and 1,25-dihydroxyvitamin D_3 to suppress PTH.
Of renal insufficiency/failure: peritoneal dialysis is the treatment of choice in infants.
Renal transplantation is the definitive treatment.

C: Hypertension, renal osteodystrophy, UTIs, and calculi.

P: Most conditions → end-stage renal failure and its associated complications. Age of onset of symptoms is associated with severity of disease.

Urinary tract infection (UTI)

D: **Symptomatic bacteriuria:**

(1) Bacteria in the urine, which is not a contaminant of urethral flora; signified by concomitant pyuria; must have both to diagnose UTI.

(2) Features of GU inflammation at particular sites: kidney (pyelonephritis), bladder (cystitis), urethra (urethritis).

Asymptomatic bacteriuria: occasionally (2% of females) bacteriuria may be discovered during investigation of another problem in an asymptomatic child. Usually does not require treatment in the older child when one would expect symptoms of dysuria/frequency.

A: **Neonates:** 70% ascending infection, 30% are of haematogenous origin.

Infants, children, adolescents: almost always ascending infection.

Organisms:

(1) Gram-negative bacteria such as *Escherichia coli* (90%), *Streptococcus faecalis*, and *Klebsiella* species from the child's faecal flora.

(2) *Proteus* (commoner in boys because it is present under the prepuce).

(3) *Staphylococcus saprophyticus* (common in adolescent girls).

(4) *Pseudomonas* (usually in children with congenital urinary tract anomalies (see chapter) or acquired renal problems, e.g. stones).

(5) Adenovirus 11 and 12 in haemorrhagic cystitis.

A/R: **Structural anomalies:** congenital GU malformations and urinary obstruction.

VUR: developmental anomaly of the vesicoureteric junctions with lateral displacement of the ureters and a shorter intramural course. 25–50% of 1st degree relatives have VUR.

E: **Neonates to infants:** highest occurrence of symptomatic UTI is at <1 year; usually due to acute pyelonephritis. M $>$ F.

Children: incidence of UTI increases again after 2 years, usually presenting as cystitis. F $>$ M.

Girls: 3–8%; have shorter urethra and closer proximity of perianal colonic organisms.

Boys: 0.5–1%.

H: **Neonates to infants:** history of unexplained fever, irritability, febrile convulsions (>6 months), vomiting/diarrhoea, poor feeding/failure to thrive, prolonged neonatal jaundice.

Children: fever with or without rigors, dysuria, frequency/retention, lethargy/anorexia, diarrhoea/vomiting, abdominal–loin pain, 2° enuresis.

E: **General:** fever, dehydration, weight loss.

Specific: loin tenderness, palpable bladder, rarely signs of CRF (see chapter).

P: **Acute pyelonephritis:** renal parenchymal infection with neutrophil infiltration; may be due to ascending ureteric infection or haematogenous spread (bacteraemia).

Chronic pyelonephritis: reflux nephropathy shows cortical scarring and clubbing of calyces.

I: **Urine collection:**

Infants: a *clean-catch* sample into a sterile pot or via suprapubic aspiration is of great importance. Adhesive plastic bags applied to the perineum may be contaminated with faecal and/or genital flora.

Children: MSU.

Urine dipstick: used as a screen for UTIs. Nitrites +/− leucocytes, blood or protein in 2 samples need to be present for diagnosis.

Urine microscopy, culture and sensitivity: $>10^5$ organisms/L of a pure growth signifies a UTI. Growth of mixed organisms in the absence of WBC signifies a contaminant. Epethelial cells also signify contamination.

Bloods: ↑WCC, U&E, ↑CRP, blood cultures (toxic child).

Radiological follow-up depends on child's age: all receive USS and DMSA.

- $<$ **1 year:** undergo MCUG independent of USS and DMSA findings.
- **Age 1–5 years:** undergo MCUG only if USS + DMSA is abnormal, or MAG3 indirect cystogram if can void on demand.
- **Age** $>$ **5 years:** MAG3 indirect cystogram if USS + DMSA is abnormal.

USS: quick, non-invasive, and involves no radiation. It identifies structural anomalies, scars, or hydronephrosis but is not good at detecting VUR.

Radioisotope scanning (DMSA): IV injection of radio-labelled DMSA is taken up by the cortical tubular cells and remains bound to them, allowing visualisation of the renal parenchyma, independent of activity in the pelvicalyceal system. The scan distinguishes areas of acute inflammation from normal renal parenchyma and gives valuable information as to whether a particular UTI has involved the kidneys or not.

MCUG: the child is catheterised and the bladder filled with contrast material. X-rays are taken as the child voids. It involves significant radiation of the genital area but is very good at detecting VUR. It should only be performed once the urine is sterile so as not to precipitate septicaemia. It is an unpleasant, traumatic investigation and so is replaced by indirect cystography once the child can void on demand.

MAG3 indirect cystogram: IV injection of MAG3, which is excreted by the kidneys. Once the whole tracer is visualised in the bladder on screening, the child is asked to void, and reflux into the ureters can readily be detected.

M: Prompt treatment is important as risk of irreversible renal damage is high especially in infants.

Treatment: oral trimethoprim. In infants and severely ill children IV cefotaxime or gentamicin may be required. Ensure good fluid intake.

Prevention: regular and complete voiding, good hygiene, avoidance of constipation, and long-term low-dose antibiotic prophylaxis (trimethoprim) for children with recurrent UTIs, reflux, scarring, and whilst awaiting investigations.

C: Chronic pyelonephritis, CRF, and hypertension (3%). VUR accounts for CRF in 20% of children and 5–10% in adults.

P: Infants who present with their 1st symptomatic UTI at age <1 year are significantly more at risk of having a recurrence; 30% risk. Preschool presentation of a UTI has a recurrence rate of 12%.

Varicella (chickenpox)

D: Contagious infectious disease caused by the DNA herpes virus varicella zoster.

A: **Antenatal:** varicella embryopathy (VE) is caused by transplacental transmission during maternal infection in 2.2% of foetuses if $<$20 weeks gestation.
Perinatal: varicella of the newborn (VON); severity depends on the time of maternal infection:

- 21–5 days before delivery: VON appears in first 4 days and there is a good prognosis.
- 5 days before delivery or 2 days after delivery: VON presents day 6–26; may be mild or severe (30% mortality).

Postnatal: transmission via the respiratory route; preterm infants are at higher risk due to lack of placental varicella IgG transfer in the 3rd trimester.
Childhood: virus enters the respiratory tract and undergoes replication in the regional lymph nodes. At 4–6 days a 1° viraemia spreads the virus to the reticuloendothelial cells primarily in the spleen and liver. At 11–24 days there is a 2° viraemia to the viscera and skin, which elicits typical skin lesions.

A: Maternal, family contact, and school contact with infected individuals.

E: 15% of pregnant women are susceptible to varicella infection. Incidence of varicella during pregnancy is 1–5/10 000. Household transmission rates are 80–90%.

H&E: **VE manifestations:**
(1) **CNS:** microcephaly, paralysis, psychomotor retardation, seizures.
(2) **Ocular:** cataracts, chorioretinitis, microphthalmia, nystagmus.
(3) **Musculoskeletal:** cicatricial dermatomal skin lesions and scarring, unilateral atrophy of a limb with scarring and paresis, rudimentary digits.

VON manifestations:
(1) **Prodrome:** poor feeding, mild pyrexia, and malaise.
(2) **Rash:** morbilliform rash in the prodrome develops into a generalised pruritic vesicular rash.

Childhood manifestations:
(1) **Prodrome:** mild pyrexia precedes skin manifestation by 1–2 days.
(2) **Rash:** appears in crops at different stages (papule, vesicle, pustule, and crust). Varicella's hallmark is the simultaneous presence of different stages and intense pruritus.
(3) **Systemic:** abdominal pain, headache, malaise, anorexia, cough, coryza, sore throat.

P: See **A**.

I: **Varicella infection is usually a clinical diagnosis.**
Specific tests: serology (varicella-specific IgM) in foetal blood, detection of varicella antigens by ELISA, virology from vesicular fluid.

M: **Conservative:** cool compresses and regular bathing to manage pruritis; discourage scratching to prevent scarring (mittens may be necessary).
Medical: acyclovir is indicated for moderate to severe disease.
VZ Ig: indicated in:
(1) Infants born to mothers with infection 5 days before delivery or 2 days after.
(2) At-risk infants ($<$28 weeks or $<$1000 g).
(3) Exposed seronegative pregnant women.
Prevention: Routine VZ immunisation is available in some countries (USA, Uruguay).

C: 1/50 cases are associated with complications, including varicella pneumonia and encephalitis.

P: In otherwise healthy children aged 1–14 years, mortality rate is 2/100 000 cases. Patients with previous VE have a higher incidence of VZ in the first 10 years of life.

D: Acyanotic congenital heart condition.

A: Defect resulting in one or more holes in the ventricular septum. 2 main types:
Perimembranous: adjacent to the tricuspid valve in the region of the membranous septum.
Muscular: defect surrounded by muscle on either side.

A/R: VSD is the most common congenital heart lesion in most chromosomal anomalies and syndromes; especially trisomy 21 (Down syndrome), 18, and 13. More common in preterm infants.

E: 4/1000 live full-term births, 5–7/1000 live preterm births; comprises 30% of all cardiac defects. It is the commonest of all cardiac defects.

H: Can be asymptomatic or symptomatic depending on the size of the defect. Symptoms for large defects include recurrent respiratory infections, symptoms of CHF; dyspnoea, palpitations (older children), and failure to thrive.

E: (1) **Small defect:** blood flowing through VSD results in a with loud harsh blowing (high-pitched) pansystolic murmur, and may be associated with a parasternal thrill.
(2) **Large defect:** parasternal heave 2° to RVH, systolic murmur is considerably softer. Additional diastolic murmur may be heard due to ↑flow through the mitral valve.

P: VSD occurs when any portion of the ventricular septum does not close after the 7th week of gestation. These defects are single or multiple. VSD can occur in any portion of the intraventricular septum including the membranous, muscular, inlet or outlet septum, or a combination of locations.

I: **CXR:** cardiomegaly with prominence of ventricles and PA with ↑pulmonary vasculature.
ECG: LVH and RVH.
Doppler + echo: for diagnostic assessment of size of defect and of CHF. Shows volume overload of left and right ventricles.

M: **Supportive management:**
(1) Antibiotic prophylaxis for dental surgery and other minor procedures is important in all septal defects.
(2) Medical treatment of associated CHF.
Surgical management:
In infancy: if child exhibits failure to thrive, CHF, or if beginnings of pulmonary hypertension.
Later repair: may be indicated if the defect fails to close and continues to cause a significant shunt. Older children with an unoperated large VSD usually require cardiac catheterisation prior to surgical closure to assess pulmonary vascular resistance; if it is too high, then it may be regarded as inoperable.

C: Infective endocarditis, CHF, pulmonary hypertension leading to Eisenmenger syndrome (cardiac failure with significant right ⟶ left shunt producing cyanosis due to pulmonary hypertension).

P: Small defects close spontaneously and have an excellent prognosis. All large defects remain open. In practice, only ~25% of children with a VSD will require surgery for it.

Visual impairment

E: Severe visual impairment affects 1/1000 births.
Developed countries: 50% genetic.
Developing countries: mainly acquired causes.

H: Lack of eye contact with parents, no responsive smiling by 6 weeks, impaired social bonding, visual inattention, random eye movements, squint, abnormal perceptual development, delays in mobility, other developmental delays.

E: May be normal if impairment is of cortical origin. However, children may lack fixation and visual tracking behaviour, or have persistent nystagmus, which is abnormal at any age. One must always assess visual acuity.

M: Maximise development of compensatory responses and available visual ability (e.g. correct any refractive errors). Advise parents on providing non-visual stimulation, ensuring safe environment, special schooling for severely visually impaired with teaching through Braille.

Strabismus (squint)

D: Abnormal alignment of both eyes. As a result, the eyes look in different directions and do not focus simultaneously on a single point.
Most commonly horizontal (convergent or divergent), but may be vertical (hypertropia – upward-looking, or hypotropia – downward-looking).

A: Failure to develop binocular vision.
Non-paralytic: more common and due to refractive error in one/both eyes.
Paralytic: rare and due to paralysis of motor nerves. When onset is rapid may be due to underlying space-occupying lesion such as a brain tumour.

A/R: Family history.

E: 4/100 children.

H: Neonates often give the appearance of having a squint because of overconvergence, but almost all correct in infancy. Strabismus is a persistent squint after 2–3 months of age (may be intermittent).

E: **Corneal light reflection test:** reflection of the light simultaneously off both corneas does not appear in the same place.
Cover test: squinting eye moves to take up fixation when normal eye covered.
Fundoscopy and neurological examination.

I: **CT/MRI brain:** if rapid onset, paralytic squint.

M: Refer all children with squints after 2–3 months to orthoptist and ophthalmologist.
Principles of treatment: develop best possible vision for each eye;

- Correct any underlying defect, e.g. cataract
- Correct refractive error with glasses
- Treat amblyopia with patch occlusion therapy if it occurs

Non-paralytic strabismus can be controlled by glasses that correct for overconvergence (long-sightedness). Congenital paralytic squints require surgery as soon as possible to enable the development of good visual function.

C: **Amblyopia:** in children, when both eyes fail to focus on the same image, the brain may learn to ignore the input from one eye. If this is allowed to continue, the eye that the brain ignores will become underdeveloped.

P: With early diagnosis and treatment the defect can usually be corrected.

Congenital cataracts

D: Opacification of lens present at birth.

A: **Familial:** usually autosomal dominant.
Congenital infection: rubella, CMV, toxoplasmosis, herpes simplex.
Drugs: corticosteroids.
Metabolic: hypocalcaemia, galactosaemia, DM.
Chromosomal: Down syndrome, Turner syndrome, trisomy 13, trisomy 18.
Idiopathic: one-third are sporadic (not associated with other disease).

E: 1/250 live births.

H: Congenital cataracts are present at birth but may not be identified until later in life. Some cataracts are static, but some are progressive. This explains why not all congenital cataracts are identified at birth.

E: Loss of red reflex, white reflex in the pupil (cataract, retinoblastoma, or ROP), photophobia.

P: Insults to developing lens fibres result in opacity.

I: Slit lamp examination. Investigate to exclude associated conditions if suspected.

M: Surgical removal of cataract, ideally before 2 months.

C: Amblyopia (if surgery delayed), strabismus, glaucoma (postsurgery).

P: Irreversibly impaired vision if untreated.

Amblyopia

D: Reduced vision in one/both eyes, without detectable cause.

A: Interference in visual input to eye during critical period (birth to 6 years) → atrophy of retinocortical pathways, resulting in loss of visual acuity. If only one eye sees clearly, it inhibits the eye with a blur; therefore amblyopia is a neurologically active process.

A/R: **Strabismus:** fixation with one eye occurs.
Anisometropia: difference in refractive power of eyes, only one eye sees clearly.
Visual deprivation: any disease blocking images reaching retina, e.g. congenital cataracts, ptosis.

E: Affects 2–3% of children. Most cases one eye, rarely both eyes.

H: Blurred vision and delay in fine motor development.

E: Visual acuity difference between eyes. Examination may be normal.

I: **CT/MRI:** to rule out other organic causes of ↓vision if examination normal.

M: Correction of any refractive error with glasses.
Patching of the 'good' eye for specific periods of the day to force brain to use the 'lazy' eye – until no more improvement occurs.
Treatment of cause if detectable, e.g. cataract.

C: Permanent loss of vision in affected eye, loss of stereopsis (two-eyed depth perception).

P: Improvement with treatment if started before 7 years.

Whooping cough (pertussis)

D: A respiratory tract infection characterised by paroxysms of coughing followed by 'whoop' (sudden massive inspiratory effort with a narrowed glottis).

A: Caused by the bacterium *Bordetella pertussis*; has an incubation period of 7–10 (up to 21) days, and is communicable for 3 weeks from the start of coughing via droplet spread.

A/R: Preterm infants, patients with underlying cardiac, pulmonary, neuromuscular, or neurological disease are at high risk for complications of pertussis (e.g. pneumonia, seizures, encephalopathy, and death).

E: **UK incidence:** 1000/year. Immunisation has decreased the risk of developing whooping cough by 80–90%. Previously, epidemics occurred in the UK every 4 years.
Peak age: 3 years. In infants <6 months it has a much higher mortality.

H&E: Pertussis has 3 stages:
Catarrhal stage: duration 1–2 weeks; indistinguishable from common URTIs with nasal congestion, rhinorrhoea, sneezing, low-grade fever, and the occasional cough. At this stage pertussis is most infectious.
Paroxysmal stage: duration 1–6 weeks; consists of paroxysms of coughing, followed in the older child by a 'whoop', with associated vomiting, dyspnoea, and possibly seizures. Infants <6 months do not have the characteristic whoop but may have apnoeic episodes.
Convalescent stage: duration weeks to months; chronic cough that becomes less paroxysmal.
Older children and adolescents: may not exhibit distinct stages. Symptoms in these patients include uninterrupted coughing, feelings of suffocation or strangulation, and headaches.

P: See **A**.

I: **Bloods:** ↑WCC, absolute lymphocytosis is common, ↑CRP, U&E.
Immunocytochemistry: direct fluorescent antibody testing of nasopharyngeal aspirates is specific but insensitive.

M: **Immunisation.**
Prophylaxis: erythromycin may be used in the catarrhal phase to decrease contagiousness of an individual or prophylactically to siblings/close contacts of a case of pertussis, especially if <1 year of age and not fully immunised.
Respiratory isolation: 5 days after starting antibiotics or until 3 weeks after the onset of the coughing spasms if the person is not receiving antibiotic treatment.
Criteria for admission:
(1) Age <6 months due to ↑mortality in this age group.
(2) Vomiting with dehydration or weight loss.
(3) Respiratory distress +/− cyanosis.
(4) Apnoea associated with paroxysms.
Notification: pertussis is a notifiable disease (CCDC).

C: **Paroxysmal cough:** may cause petechiae and conjunctival haemorrhages. Lack of intake may cause dehydration and weight loss.
Seizures (3%): if encephalopathy follows; one-third die, one-third remain neurologically impaired, one-third recover fully.
2° infections: otitis media, bronchiectasis, and pneumonia (main cause of pertussis-related deaths).

P: Usually lasts 6–8 weeks; however, a prolonged illness may occur ('100-day cough'). There is significant morbidity and mortality in infants <6 months in whom apnoea associated with paroxysms may cause sudden death.

APPENDICES

What is the difference between adult and paediatric consultations?

(1) History is often given mainly by third party; and may be modified by parent perception or interpretation.
(2) Extra components to history: pregnancy and birth, feeding history in infancy, immunisations, growth, developmental milestones, behaviour, and schooling.
(3) History and examination are modified according to the child's age and development.

Important points to note before taking a history:

(1) Check if you know the child's name, age, and gender.
(2) Introduce yourself; explain who you are and your role in the child's care.
(3) Remember to address questions to the child if appropriate.
(4) Establishing a good rapport with the child and family is essential.
(5) Make toys available. Observe how the child interacts with parents and siblings.

Presenting complaint:

(1) It is important to find out what prompted referral to a doctor.
(2) What do the parents think or fear may be wrong?
(3) Use open questions such as 'What is worrying you about Tom?'
(4) Let the parent tell the story of the presenting problem without interruptions.
(5) Was the child completely well beforehand? Have there been any foreign travel/sick contacts?
(6) Avoid using medical jargon.
(7) Use the child's and parents' own words, and make sure the words they use, e.g. wheeze, mean the same thing to you.

General enquiry:

(1) Is the child active and lively as usual? Any recent change in behaviour or personality?
(2) Does the child have the same appetite as usual: eating and drinking usual amounts?
(3) Is the child growing/gaining weight at a normal rate?
(4) Any fevers, rashes, lumps, pruritis?

Systems review if indicated:

(1) **Cardiovascular:** cyanosis, exercise tolerance.
(2) **Respiratory:** grunting, wheeze, cough (nocturnal/chronic), sputum production.
(3) **GI:** jaundice (duration/onset), diarrhoea, vomiting, stool frequency, abdominal pain.
(4) **GU:** how often is the nappy wet, haematuria, dysuria (older child), sexual development.
(5) **Neuromuscular:** feeding ability, abnormal movements, seizures, headaches, hearing/vision ability.
(6) **ENT:** noisy breathing, ear discharge, sore throat, teething.

Past medical history:

(1) ***In utero*:** how was the pregnancy? Use of medication, alcohol intake, and smoking in pregnancy. Rh disease, maternal rubella, other viral infections *in utero*.

(2) **At birth:** gestation at birth, type of delivery, use of forceps/Caesarean, birth weight, condition of infant at birth (APGAR scores), need for medical intervention, admission to SCBU, ventilation.
(3) **As a neonate:** jaundice, fits, fevers, feeding problems, weight gain.
(4) **Childhood:** operations, illnesses, hospital admission, accidents, injuries.

Immunisations:

Take time to go through what has been administered and compare this to the recommended schedule.

Growth and development:

(1) Plot growth measurements on appropriate length/height, weight, and head circumference charts.
(2) Find out usual daily pattern of food intake (breastfeeding/types of formula feed, intake pattern later).
(3) **Infants and toddlers:** use 'screening' questions that determine developmental progress at hallmark ages for each of the 4 major areas of development: gross motor control; fine motor and vision; speech, language, and hearing; social behaviour and play.
(4) **Older children:** ask about progress in nursery/school, and parent assessment in comparison with siblings/peers.

Drug history:

(1) Past and present medications plus OTC medication and alternative therapies.
(2) Drug intolerances, adverse reactions, and true allergies.

Family history:

(1) Draw a family tree over 3 generations, age of parent and siblings, medical problems in the family.
(2) Consanguinity?
(3) Positive family history for atopy, DM, seizures, jaundice, renal disease, TB.

Social history:

(1) Who lives in the household and who provides most of the child's care?
(2) Does the child live in more than one household? Marital separation/stresses?
(3) Parental occupation? Economic status? Do they receive financial allowances? Housing?
(4) Factors that might adversely affect child's health, e.g. household members smoking? (very important).
(5) Check whether child is on the Child Protection Register.

Closing questions:

(1) Is there anything else that is worrying you?
(2) Is there anything else I should know or anything I have forgotten to ask you?

Neonatal Life Support algorithm

Dry the infant, remove any wet clothing and cover

Initial assessment at birth; start the clock
Assess: colour, tone, breathing, HR.

If not breathing

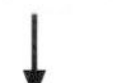

Control the airway with head in neutral position

Support the breathing
5 inflation breaths (each 2–3 s in duration).
Confirm a response: ↑ in HR or visible chest movement.

If there is no response
Check head position and apply jaw thrust.
5 inflation breaths.
Confirm a response with ↑ in HR or visible chest movement.

If there is still no response
(1) Enlist a 2nd person to help with airways control and repeat inflated breaths.
(2) Inspect the oropharynx under direct vision to assess if suction is needed, repeat inflation breaths.
(3) Insert oropharyngeal Guedel airways and repeat inflation breaths.
(4) *Consider intubation*.
Confirm a response: ↑ in HR or visible chest movement.

When the chest is moving
Continue the ventilation breaths if no spontaneous breathing.

Check the HR
If the heart is not detectable or slow (<60 bpm and not ↑).

Start chest compressions
First confirm chest movement; if chest not moving, return to airways.
3 chest compressions to 1 breath for 30 s.

↓

Reassess HR
If improving, stop chest compressions and continue ventilation if not breathing.
If the heart is still slow, continue ventilation and chest compressions.
Consider venous access and drugs at this stage.

Formal assessment of the neonate at birth

All neonates are graded with an APGAR score at birth.
This is a scoring system (out of 10) based on:
A: Activity.
P: Pulse.
G: Grimacing/reflex irritability on suctioning.
A: Appearance.
R: Respiratory effort of the baby.

- **7–10** is considered normal.
- **4–7** might require some resuscitative measures.
- < **3** requires immediate resuscitation.

Sign		0 points	1 point	2 points
A	Activity	No movement	Arms and legs flexed	Active movement
P	Pulse	Absent	< 100 bpm	> 100 bpm
G	Grimacing/reflex irritability	No response	Grimace	Pulls away
A	Appearance	Blue/pale all over	Extremities pale	Normal colour
R	Respiratory effort	Absent	Slow/irregular gasps	Normal rate/effort

APGARs are not useful specific predictors of neurodevelopmental outcome except when extremely and persistently low, or when accompanied by deep acidaemia. Even with APGARs as low as 3 at 10 min, 80% of infants of normal birth weight are free of major disability by early school age (The National Institute of Health, National Collaborative Perinatal Project).

Foetal scalp/umbilical cord blood: may be required to identify metabolic acidosis and the necessity for emergency Caesarean section (pH < 7.25). APGARs are better predictors than cord pH as some babies come out screaming with a pH of 6.9 and are fine, whereas the floppy, unresponsive baby at 10 min with a normal pH is much more at risk.

Prognosis: in the last 20 years despite all the changes in obstetric practice including CTGs, foetal scalp bloods sampling, although the neonatal mortality rate has declined, the rates of cerebral palsy have remained static at 2/1000 live births.

Measurements: Weight, length, and head circumference should be recorded on a centile chart.

General observation: Undress infant for the examination.

General neurological state: Can be observed whilst undressing the infant; neuromuscular tone, degree of activity, irritability, and lethargy.

Primitive newborn reflexes: Moro's reflex (startle reflex) and the grasp reflex.

Colour: Jaundice, pallor, plethora, or cyanosis.

Dysmorphic features: Pattern recognition for various syndromes.

Limitation of movement: May indicate deep tissue injury, e.g. fractured clavicle or humerus during labour.

Skin

Vernix: White substance that protects the foetus from overhydration.

Lanugo: Fine downy hair covering the skin of the shoulders, upper arms, and thighs.

Petechiae: Small haemorrhagic skin lesions, they may be benign on the face but if on the trunk may indicate thrombocytopenia.

Milia: Small sebaceous cysts that occur particularly over the nose.

Vesicles: Uncommon but may be the first signs of infection (e.g. HSV).

Erythema toxicum: Vesiculomacular rash with an erythematous base that is often widespread, the vesicles contain eosinophils.

Pustules: May appear at birth in congenital candidal infection or may appear later with *Staphylococcus aureus* infection.

Birthmarks

- Naevus flammeus; stork bites.
- Mongolian spots; pigmented naevus often large and on the lower back.
- Port-wine stain; deep vascular naevus may be found in the distribution of a division of the trigeminal nerve. (associated Sturge–Weber syndrome).
- Strawberry naevus; raised naevus that becomes larger then regresses spontaneously by 3 years.
- Pigmented naevus; familial and often large and hairy.

Hands

Polydactyly: Excessive number of digits/tags.

Lymphoedema: Hands or feet suggestive of Turner syndrome.

Simian creases: Present unilaterally in 5% of the population, if present bilaterally may indicate presence of Down syndrome (look for other associated features).

Limbs

Achondroplasia: Short-limbed dwarfism is associated with a reduction in the length of the proximal segment of the limb relative to the distal segment.

Arthrogryposis: Restriction of joint movements; may suggest connective tissue defects.

Head

Microcephalus: Head circumference < 3rd percentile; associated with Down syndrome, intrauterine infection, symmetrical IUGR.

Macrocephalus: Head circumference > 97th percentile; associated with ↑ ICP 2° to hydrocephalus, but may be benign 2° to tall stature.

Bradycephalus: Squareness of the head when viewed from above; may indicate Down syndrome.

Plagiocephalus: Elongation of the head; may indicate premature fusion of one of the skull sutures.

Fontanelle: Anterior and posterior should be palpated for tension and size.

Haematomas: 2 different types can occur; cephalhaematoma that occurs beneath the periosteum and tissue haematomas that occur spontaneously or as a result of instrumental delivery.

Encephalocele: Caused by the failure of closure of the neural tube and may be present in the midline of the head. Another neural tube defect is spina bifida that results in a lower spine lesion.

Face

Ears: Size, form, and position; patency of the external auditory meatus. Look for pre- or post-auricular skin tags (targeted neonatal hearing test required).

Eyes: The red reflex should be sought (bright red view though the retina is normal), the pupil is white with congenital cataracts or retinoblastomas.

Mouth

Cleft lip/palate: Unilateral or bilateral. Elicit by palpation and visualisation of the hard and soft palates.

Tongue

Macroglossia: Beckwith–Wiedemann syndrome (hypertrophy of limbs, and neonatal hypoglycaemia).

Nose

Choanal atresia: Abnormal membrane covers the nasopharynx, which causes airways obstruction.

Neck

Lateral masses: May be a cystic hygroma or branchial cyst (soft fluctuant swellings that transluminate).

Midline masses: Most likely to be a goitre.

Lateral fistulae: Remnants of the branchial arch.

Thorax

Respiratory rate: > 60/min is tachypnoea.

Signs of respiratory distress: Recession; intercostal/subcostal/sternal/sub-sternal, use of the accessory muscles of respiration, expiratory grunting, or nasal flaring.

Asymmetry of the hemithoraces: Pneumothorax or a congenital heart defect with cardiac enlargement.

Breast: Engorgement is common, widely spaced nipples may indicate Turner syndrome.

Cardiovascular

Pulse rate: Normally 100–160 bpm felt in the antecubital fossa.

Femoral pulses: Weak femoral pulse (COA), strong femoral pulse (PDA).

Auscultation: Innocent flow murmurs (in 30%); usually soft blowing systolic murmur localised to left sternal edge with no radiation and normal heart sounds in an asymptomatic patient. See chapters on congenital cardiac anomalies for details on various pathological murmurs.

Abdomen

Shape: Distension may indicate intestinal obstruction; 'scaphoid' (concave) is indicative of a diaphragmatic hernia.

Hepatomegaly: Normal liver may be palpated up to 4 cm below the costal margin. Hepatomegaly may occur in infections (EBV/CMV), malignancy, inborn errors of metabolism, or haemolytic anaemia (e.g. sickle-cell).

Splenomegaly: Intrauterine infection or underlying haematological condition.

Umbilical cord: Should be clean and contain 3 vessels.

Hernial orifices: Visual inspection or palpation.

Genitalia

Females: Prominent labia minora are normal, a mucoid vaginal discharge is common in the first few weeks, and an imperforate hymen may also be present. The site of the anus should be visualised to exclude imperforate anus.

Males: Urethral meatus should be visualised at the tip of the penis, not the underside (hypospadias). Feel for testes in the scrotum.

Hips

DDH: Barlow/Ortolani test. Abduction may be limited and a displaced hip relocates with an audible 'clunk'. 'Clicky' hips are usually normal; reflecting cartilaginous/ligamentous involvement.

Feet

Positional talipes: Feet often remain in *in utero* position, but can be dorsi-flexed to touch the front of the lower leg (requires physiotherapy input).

Talipes equinovarus (club-foot): Entire foot is inverted and supinated and the forefoot is adducted. This position is fixed and needs to be corrected surgically.

Toes: May be supernumerary or absent.

Breastfeeding vs. bottle-feeding

FOR THE CHILD

Advantages of breastfeeding vs. bottle-feeding	Disadvantages of breastfeeding vs. bottle-feeding
Nutritional: (1) Protein, lipid, iron, and other vitamins/minerals, e.g. vitamin D; right quantity and better bioavailability. (2) Appropriate electrolyte content (e.g. sodium) important due to immaturity of renal concentrating system. (3) Colostrum (first few days): protein and Ig, important for establishment of lactobacilli in the gut. (4) Polyunsaturated fatty acids are beneficial in neuronal and retinal development. (5) Ensures right concentration of nutrients; formula feeds may be too concentrated/dilute. **Humoral immunological transmission:** (1) Secretory IgA contributes to mucosal immune barrier. (2) Bifidus factor promotes growth of *Lactobacillus bifidus* that inhibits growth of GI pathogens. (3) Lysozyme lyses bacterial cell walls. (4) Lactoferrin binds iron necessary for replication of *Escherichia coli* and other bacteria. (5) Interferon is an antiviral agent. **Cellular immunological transmission:** macrophages, T and B lymphocytes, polymorphs. **Sterility of breast milk:** reduced GI infections especially in developing countries. ↓**Risk and severity of disease:** GORD, IBD, NEC, SIDS (not proven). **Total sensory experience (all 5 senses).** **Bonding with mother.**	**Contraindications:** (1) Maternal active untreated TB, brucellosis, or recently acquired syphilis. (2) HIV-positive mothers (UK guidelines); in developing countries HIV-positive mothers are still encouraged to breastfeed as the protection from life-threatening gastroenteritis outweighs risk of ↑transmisson rate of HIV. (3) Metabolic disorders in the baby, e.g. maple syrup urine disease. (4) Maternal drugs: antithyroid (carbimazole), antimetabolic (methotrexate), chemotherapy, lithium, and tetracycline. **Nutritional:** Low in vitamin K; required to prevent haemorrhagic disease of the newborn. **Preventable negative aspects:** (1) Prolonged exclusive breastfeeding to >6 months may result in poor weight gain. (2) Maternal transmission of hepatitis B; mothers can breastfeed once the child is immunised. (3) Potential transmission of maternal substance: smoking, alcohol, illicit drugs.

FOR THE MOTHER

Advantages of breastfeeding vs. bottle-feeding	Disadvantages of breastfeeding vs. bottle-feeding
Psychological: helps mother to establish an intimate, loving relationship with her baby. **Practicalities:** (1) Breast milk is sterile and free. (2) Is at the correct temperature. (3) Avoids preparation needed for formula feed.	**Preventable negative aspects;** with good support and advice the following are preventable: (1) Difficulty initialising breastfeeding and failure to fix can cause emotional upset for the mother. (2) Local infection due to poor management: painful, cracked nipples, mastitis, or breast abscesses. **Work environment:** there may be no convenient place to breastfeed.
Reduction in postpartum haemorrhage: oxytocin released contracts uterine vessels.	
Reduction in disease: (1) Premenopausal breast cancer. (2) Ovarian cancer. (3) Osteoporosis.	
Return to pre-pregnant weight sooner.	
Contraceptive, especially in developing countries.	

There is no better nutrition for infants than breastfeeding.

1989 WHO/UNICEF Ten Steps to Successful Breastfeeding:

(1) Written breastfeeding policy that is routinely communicated to all health care professionals.
(2) Train all health care staff in skills necessary to implement this policy.
(3) Inform all pregnant mothers about the benefits and management of breastfeeding.
(4) Help mothers initiate breastfeeding within 1/2 h of delivery.
(5) Show mothers how to breastfeed, and how to maintain lactation even if separated from their infants.
(6) Give newborn infants no food or drink other than breast milk unless medically indicated.
(7) Practise 'rooming-in' (allow mothers and infants to remain together), 24 h a day.
(8) Encourage unrestricted breastfeeding.
(9) Give no artificial teats or pacifiers (dummies) to breastfeeding infants.
(10) Foster the establishment of breastfeeding, support groups and refer mothers to them on discharge from hospital or clinic.

Lapse in breastfeeding: 71% of mothers in the UK start breastfeeding (UK Infant feeding 2000); however, this reduces to 52% at 2 weeks and 39% at 6 weeks after delivery. The reasons mothers give up are:

(1) Pain and discomfort from mastitis, breast abscess, cracked nipples, breast thrush.
(2) Concerns that they are not producing enough milk and stressed by 'test' weighing.
(3) Returning to work, inadequate facilities for breastfeeding, attitudes in the work environment.

Maternal support: mothers need to be encouraged to continue breastfeeding by education about the benefits both the mother and the child will receive. They need to have access to appropriate support such as midwives and health care professionals, especially during the initial establishment of breastfeeding and there needs to be better provision for breastfeeding in the work environment. Do not test weigh.

Formula feeds: are an alternative to breast milk where it is contraindicated or decided against based on modified cow's milk. Unmodified cow's milk contains too much protein, sodium, potassium, calcium, phosphorus, and inadequate iron, vitamins, and essential fatty acids.

Properties of standard formula feed:
Protein: contains cow's protein modified by addition of whey to modify whey/casein ratio.
Fats: from vegetable oils with saturated and unsaturated fatty acids in similar ratio to breast milk.
Carbohydrates: from lactose.
Vitamins and minerals: are supplemented.

Principles of bottle-feeding:

(1) The infant's appetite should determine the volume and number of feeds, initially (≈150 ml/kg/24 h).
(2) Use safe water and sterilised utensils and equipment.

(3) Ensure correct preparation with accurate measurement of powder for formula reconstitution.

Cow's milk: full fat cow's milk can be introduced as the main milk source from 12 months of age. Prior to this it may cause microscopic GI blood loss. Reduced fat milk can be introduced after 5 years.

Soya milk formulae: commonly and inappropriately used for:
(1) Suspected cow's milk protein intolerance; 30% will also develop clinical intolerance to soya.
(2) Lactose intolerance; best to use lactose-modified formulae.
(3) Prevent allergies; no evidence of protection with soya.

Risks: soy formulae have a higher aluminium content and phytates that inhibit absorption of minerals, especially calcium. The impact of phyto-oestrogen exposure (in the form of isoflavones) in infancy has been controversial of late, as these bind to oestrogen receptors and may exert tissue-specific effects.

Indications: soy formula is indicated children with galactosaemia and in vegan families who will not use cow's milk.

Weaning: between 4 and 6 months infants have the muscle tone and maturity of the digestive system to begin eating solid foods; however, the WHO advise exclusive breastfeeding till 6 months. WHO also recommends breastfeeding alongside supplementation with solid food until the age of 2. The term weaning can be misleading as it implies the cessation of breastfeeding.

First foods: soft or puréed food such as iron-fortified cereal foods followed by fruits and vegetables. Meats and poultry can be introduced from 7 months when children begin to chew along with custard, cheese, and yoghurt.

Advanced Life Support algorithm

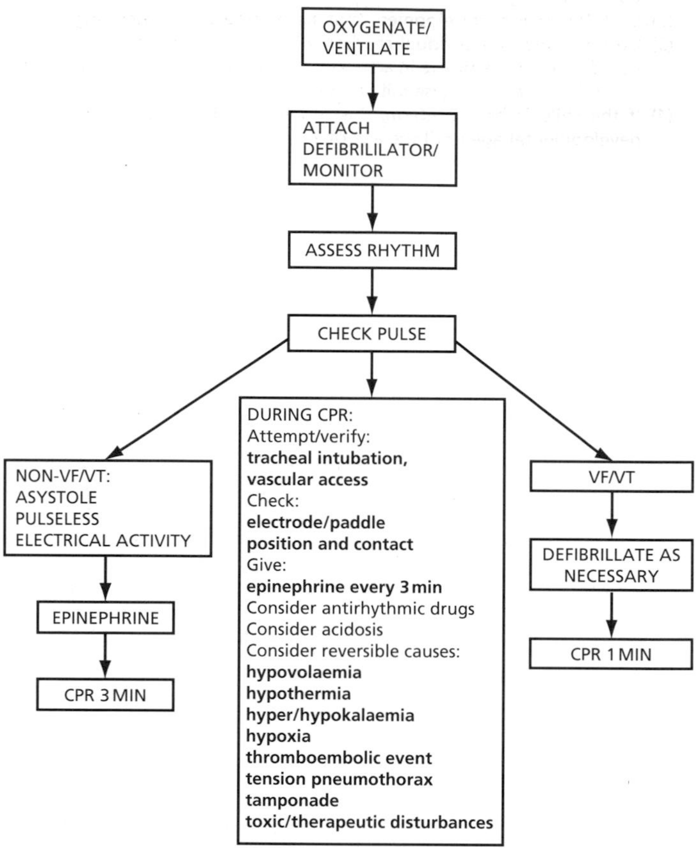

Differences between adult and paediatric resuscitation

Airway:

- Position head to open airways in a neutral position (jaw thrust manoeuvre if still obstructed).
- Immobilise cervical spine if trauma related with collar, sandbags, and tape. If child becomes combative a hard collar should be applied and no attempt made to immobilise the head.

Breathing: most paediatric arrests are primarily respiratory.

Circulation:

- Feel pulse at femoral/brachial or carotid (depending on age of child).
- Commence external cardiac compressions if absent or less than 60 bpm in infants.
- Rate of compressions:
  (1) 0–1 year – 120/min.
  (2) 1–5 years – 100/min.
  (3) >5 years – 80/min.
- Compression/respiration ratio 5 : 1.

Monitoring: ECG, BP, pulsoximetry (same as adult).

Venous access: antecubital fossa or external jugular. If unsuccessful, establish intraosseus access.

Key principles:

(1) Always take a longitudinal approach in time when assessing a child's developmental progress.

(2) Look for areas of development that are outside the normal range.

(3) Do not compare individual children with 'normal' milestones as these are based on the median age in achievement. Therefore 50% of children will by definition not meet these milestones.

(4) If the child is born preterm, this should be allowed for when assessing developmental age until the age of 2.

Developmental abilities and warning signs* at ages often used in assessment.

Normal ranges	Gross motor control	Fine motor and vision	Speech, language and hearing	Social behaviour and play
2–4 months	***Asymmetry/absence of primitive reflexes.** Moro's, grasp, stepping, and atonic neck reflex. Lifts head briefly when sitting up.	***Persistent squint.** Stares intently. Follows moving object or face by turning the head in 90° arc.	***No response to loud noises.** Stills to mother's voice. Startles to loud noise. Squeals with pleasure.	***Not smiling.** Smiles and coos responsively.
6–9 months	***Persistent primitive reflexes.** Lifts head up from prone with weight on hands, can roll over. Sits without support. Crawls, can pull to stand, can weight bear on legs when standing.	***Persistent hand preference at $>$ 6/12.** Palmar grasp (6/12). Index approach (9/12). Transfers from hand to hand/mouth (7/12). Pincer grip (9/12). Fixes and can follow small objects.	***Reduced response. Absence of babble.** Responds to name. 'Ma, Da' at 6/12. 'Mama, Dada' at 9/12. Uses sounds indiscriminately. Understands 'No'. Turns to soft sounds out of sight.	***Absent or slow social responses.** Puts food in mouth. Chews biscuit. Plays peak-a-boo. Shows object to mother at 9/12. Pats mirror image. Interest in people. Awareness of strangers.
10–12 months	***Immature grasp/asymmetry of grasp.** **No sitting or weight bearing.** Reaches behind. Cruises round furniture. Walks alone but unsteadily with broad gait and hands apart.	***Holds objects close up to eyes.** Throws objects. Watches them fall. Picks up crumbs from carpet. Pincer grip. Bangs bricks together.	***No frequent babble by 10/12.** Understands some words. Uses 'Mama, Dada' discriminately. Uses 2–3 other words. Shakes head for 'No'.	***Constant mouthing.** Comes when called. Lets go on request. Finds hidden objects. Waves bye-bye. Drinks from cup.
13–18 months	***Not walking: consider myotonic dystrophy.** Walks well, carries toys, climbs stairs, climbs into chair.	***Absent pincer grip.** Neat pincer grip: picks up threads, pins. Scribbles using fist. Builds tower of 3 – 4 × 1″ (2.5 cm) cubes. Turns 2 pages at a time.	***Drools.** **No words. Not understanding commands.** Points to parts of body on request. Obeys single commands. Echoes speech: 6 words, jargons.	***Not interacting appropr-iately.** Lifts cups, drinks, and puts down safely, spoon-feeds self. Pulls at dirty nappy. Domestic mimicry, finger-feeding. Protodeclarative pointing, symbolic play.

Developmental abilities and warning signs* at ages often used in assessment (cont.)

Normal ranges	Gross motor control	Fine motor and vision	Speech, language and hearing	Social behaviour and play
2–2.5 years	***Unsteady on feet.** Runs, kicks ball, jumps on the spot, walks down stairs 2 feet per tread.	***Parental concerns.** Turns 1 page at a time. Imitates a straight vertical and horizontal line and a circle. Unscrews lids. Builds tower of 6–8 × 1″ cubes.	***Lack of understanding of speech.** **No phrases by 2.5 yrs.** Phrases of 2–3 words, gives names, naming games, 50+ words.	***Parental concerns.** Plays alone. Tantrums, demanding. Dry by day. Puts on shoes and pants. Turns door-handles. Uses spoon and fork. Interested in other children.
3–3.5 years	***Clumsy (motor cause).** Stands on one leg for a few seconds. Peddles tricycle. Adult ascent of stairs. Jumps off bottom step.	***Clumsy (visual cause).** Mature pen grasp, copies + and O. Correctly matches 2+ colours. Tower of 9 × 1″ cubes.	***No phrases.** **Echolalia.** Gives full name, sex. Counts to 10 by rote. Uses plurals. Understands prepositions. 3 to 5-word sentences.	***Persistent daytime wetting/soiling.** Uses toilet unassisted except wiping bottom. Dresses and undresses with minimum assistance. 'Why' questions. Nursery rhymes. Uses knife and fork. Plays with peers.
4–5 years	***Any parental concerns.** 4 years: climbs trees and ladders. Enjoys ball games. 5 years: hops, skips, jumps 3 steps, catches a ball.	***Any parental concerns.** Matches 4 colours. 5 years: copies cross, square, and triangle. 4 years: 3 steps with 6 cubes. 5 years: 4 steps with 10 cubes. Draws a recognisable man.	***Unintelligible/ungrammatical speech.** **Unable to give name and address.** 4 years: counts to 10. 5 years: counts to 20. Transient stammer from urgency to speak is common. Asks meaning of abstract words.	***Socially isolated/bullied.** Wipes own bottom. Eats using knife and fork. Dresses unsupervised except for tie, laces. Imaginative play. Separates from mother.

* Warning signs.

Immunisation schedule

The single most useful thing that doctors can do to improve child health

UK National Immunisation Programme 2000

Birth <12 h	1 month	2 months	3 months	4 months	6–12 months	12–15 months	18 months	24 months	4–6 years	11–12 years	14–16 years
BCG *at risk only*		DPT	DPT	DPT					DT	BCG *if negative tuberculin*	DT
Hep B *at risk only*	Hep B *at risk only*				Hep B *at risk only*						
		Hib	Hib	Hib							
		Men C	Men C	Men C					*Men C*		*Men C*
		OPV	OPV	OPV					OPV		OPV
						MMR			MMR		

KEY

UK immunisation schedule

BCG: bacille Calmette–Guérin; live attenuated *Mycobacteria bovis* vaccine.
At risk = TB in the family within last 6 months.
DT: diphtheria, tetanus; inactivated toxins.
DPT: diphtheria, pertussis, tetanus; inactivated toxins.
Hep B: hepatitis B; recombinant proteins of surface antigen.
At risk = mother is HBsAg positive.
Polio (OPV): live oral polio vaccine; live attenuated virus.
MMR: measles, mumps, rubella; live attenuated viruses.
Hib: conjugated *Haemophilus influenzae* b vaccine; polysaccharide capsule of the inactivated organism conjugated with a protein.
Men C: conjugated meningococcal C vaccine; polysaccharide capsule of the inactivated organism conjugated with a protein.
Men C: convenient times at which missed doses can be administered.

Other vaccines

Immunisation schedule in the USA: pneumococcal vaccine (2, 4, 6 months and booster 12–15 months), varicella vaccine (12–18 months).
At-risk infants: hepatitis A vaccine (2–16 years in selected areas), pneumococcal influenza vaccine in Down syndrome, congenital cardiac anomalies, CF.
Being tested: meningitis B vaccine.

General notes:

- Vaccination should be postponed if the child has an acute febrile illness (>38%).
- Do not give live vaccines if there is a 1° immunodeficiency disorder, or if the child is taking oral steroids.
- Do not give BCG in children with HIV, but give all other vaccines.
- Vaccines may have mild side-effects; pain at site of injection, fever +/− rash after incubation period.

MMR note: area of controversy in recent times:

- Originated in 1998 with a case report by Andrew Wakefield published in the *Lancet* – in a study of 12 children he proposed a link between the MMR vaccine and autism and inflammatory bowel disease.
- Since the original study no evidence of a link has been found by the Medical Research Council review (1998), a large 14-year Finnish study (2001), WHO (2001/2003), Institute of Medicine (2002), and 2 studies by Taylor *et al*. (*Lancet* 1999; BMJ 2002).
- Despite this vaccination rates are falling and the incidence of measles, mumps, and rubella is rising.
- Single vaccinations are not recommended as there is not enough research into their use, and are likely to be more harmful due to delay in vaccination or poor completion (6 injections).
- There has been no link substantiated between the MMR vaccination, autism and inflammatory bowel disease.

Child health surveillance/promotion

1° prevention: usually GP- and health visitor-mediated.

Aims:

(1) High levels of immunisation of all children.
(2) BCG, hepatitis B, hepatitis A, pneumococcal, varicella, and influenza vaccines in high-risk groups.
(3) Education on SIDS (e.g. 'back to sleep' campaign, avoiding smoky environments, overheating).
(4) Education on inadvertent injury (including poisoning).

Screening procedures:

(1) Following birth: see examination of the newborn appendix.
(2) 5–6 days: Guthrie's test (blood spot test) for PKU, congenital hypothyroidism and CF.
(3) 1 week: new automated hearing test using otoacoustic emissions and/or auditory brainstem-evoked responses.
(4) 6–8 weeks: enquiry about parental concerns and general physical examination for:
    - Height, weight, and head circumference on centile chart.
    - DDH.
    - CHD.
    - Hypertension.
    - Abnormalities of the genitalia and ensure testicular descent.
    - Cataracts and squints.
(5) 6–9 months: height, weight, and head circumference on centile chart. Hearing test if not tested at 1 week (see Hearing impairment).
(6) 4–5 years (pre-school): height and weight on centile chart, impedance audiometry hearing test, visual screening test (Snellen chart).

Growth monitoring: routine measurement of height, weight, and head circumference recorded on the 9 centile growth charts to detect:

(1) Impaired growth: hypothyroidism, GH deficiency, Turner syndrome, intracranial tumours, bone dysplasias (see Short stature).
(2) Failure to thrive (see chapter).
(3) Excessive growth: thyrotoxicosis, congenital adrenal hyperplasia, Marfan syndrome, precocious puberty.

Immunisations: (see chapter for full immunisation schedule):

- 2–4 months: 3× DPT, Hib, men C, polio vaccines.
- 12–15 months: MMR vaccine.
- 4–6 years: MMR, DT, and polio booster vaccines.
- 14–16 years: DT and polio booster vaccines.

Personal child health records: parents hold this main record of their child's health and development so as to encourage a partnership between health care professionals and parents.

Contents:

(1) Summary of birth, vitamin K administration, neonatal examination.
(2) Immunisation record (date, site, who administered).
(3) 9 centile national growth charts.
(4) Information on feeding (at 4, 8, 12,16 weeks).

Sure Start

'Sure Start' is a UK government-funded programme for young children living in underprivileged environments. Voluntary agencies, community groups, and local parents work as partners to improve the outcome of these children. Each programme covers around 750 children under the age of 4, involves home visits to new parents, quality play, childcare and enhanced health advice.

Status epilepticus*

D: Seizures lasting for > 30 minutes or repeated seizures without intervening consciousness.

M:

Airway: clear and stabilise

Breathing: high flow O_2 via face mask, measure saturations.
Circulation: IV access (or intraosseus), measure pulse and BP.
Blood glucose (BM): if blood glucose is < 3 mmol/L, give IV dextrose.

Immediate IV access

Step 1. Lorazepam: 0.1 mg/kg IV over 30–60 s

↓ 10 min ↓

Step 2. Lorazepam: 0.1 mg/kg IV over 30–60 s

↓ 10 min

No IV access

Diazepam: 0.5 mg/kg PR

↓ 10 min ↓ (or ↙ IV access → Step 2)

Paraldehyde: 0.4 ml/kg PR

↓ 10 min

Get senior help

Step 3. Phenytoin infusion: 18 mg/kg IV over 20 min.
If on phenytoin as regular anti-convulsant, give phenobartitone 20 mg/kg IV over 10 min instead.
Can use intraosseus route.
Give paraldehyde 0.4 ml/kg PR if not already given.
Call anaesthetist/PICU.

Step 4. If child still in status 20 min after commencement of Step 3, rapid induction of anaesthesia using thiopentone.

Transfer to PICU

Step 5. Empirical IV antibiotics/antivirals:

- Ceftriaxone.
- Erythromycin/clarithromycin if penicillin-allergic.
- Acyclovir.

Think of a cause

Febrile convulsion, change of medication, idiopathic epilepsy, encephalitis, meningitis, poisoning, metabolic disorder, hypoxia, acute cerebral trauma.

Mandatory investigations

Blood glucose, calcium, phosphate, magnesium, FBC, U&E, ABG, ECG.

Optional investigations

Toxicology, septic screen (beware of raised ICP and consider carefully if LP is necessary), LFTs, metabolic screen, coagulation, CXR, cranial imaging.

* Modified from BPNA 2000 guidelines.